Digital Healthcare
THE ESSENTIAL GUIDE

**DR RUTH CHAMBERS, MARC SCHMID,
JAYNE BIRCH-JONES**

Otmoor Publishing
Oxford

Otmoor Publishing Ltd
Oxford OX5 2RD
United Kingdom

British Library Cataloguing Publication Data

A catalogue record for this book is available from the British Library.

ISBN-13 978 1 910303 06 1

Cover design by Cox Design, Witney, Oxfordshire, UK

Cartoons by John Byrne. http://johnbyrnecartoons.com

Typeset and designed by Darkriver Design, Auckland, New Zealand
Printed by Printondemand-Worldwide.com

Contents

Foreword   v
Preface   vii
Disclaimer   viii
About the authors   ix

Part One: What is digital healthcare?   1

1   Where we are now with technology enabled care and services   3
    Dr Ruth Chambers

2   Telehealth   23
    Dr Ruth Chambers

3   Why assistive technology should be a key part of health and social
    care services   41
    Richard Haynes

4   Applying telecare and assistive technology in practice   57
    Jim Ellam

5   Telemedicine and video or Skype consultations: gaining benefits,
    minimising risks and barriers, and overcoming challenges   69
    Marc Schmid

6   Apps: the future is mobile   93
    Marc Schmid

7   Use social media? Get the benefits but minimise risks   105
    Marc Schmid

Part Two: Making digital healthcare happen   121

8   Patient and public perspectives:
    listen and communicate well   123
    Jayne Birch-Jones, Dr Ruth Chambers

9   Making digital delivery happen in health and social care: at an organisational level   133

Dr Ruth Chambers

10   Making digital delivery happen as an individual manager or practitioner: adopting established technology and innovation   147

Dr Ruth Chambers

11   Commissioning, implementing and mainstreaming technology enabled care services   159

Jayne Birch-Jones

12   Managing risks of technology enabled care services   175

Jayne Birch-Jones, Dr Ruth Chambers

13   Overcoming resistance and maximising opportunities for the adoption of technology enabled care services   187

Lisa Taylor

14   Including technology in the delivery of person-centred, integrated care   197

Dr Ruth Chambers

Part Three: Moving digital healthcare on   205

15   Learning about technology enabled care services: so improving uptake   207

Dr Ruth Chambers

16   Evaluation of technology enabled care services   229

Dr Lizzie Cottrell, Dr Ruth Chambers

17   The future: what will remote delivery of healthcare look like in five years' time?   245

John Uttley, Ciaron Hoye, Jayne Birch-Jones

Index   261

Foreword

Three years ago, I travelled to the United States with one of the authors and some of the contributors to *Digital Healthcare: the essential guide* on a National Health Service Leadership Exchange with the US Department of Veterans Affairs. Day after day we saw evidence of the power of making digital connections between service providers and service users: our lives would never be the same again!

In this guide Ruth, Marc and Jayne present an accumulated wealth of knowledge from authors who are embedded at the front line of health and care. The book offers a powerful case for accelerating the potential of digital health, which enables a transformational health and care information exchange that was previously impossible. It captures the aim of value-based care, the goal of which is to lower healthcare costs and improve quality and outcomes. As a proponent of personally held healthcare records during my 19 years of working with patients, and having run a digitally enabled home-visiting optician service, it is fantastic to see the progress that has been made. Digital technology is making it much easier for professionals to share knowledge and build understanding and confidence in the lives of the people they are serving. Convenience is a major benefit as well, and with trends showing that the public expect to be able to have the expediency of remote monitoring and consultations through apps and online, there is every reason to harness digital health.

This is an immensely practical book cum workbook which has been missing on the market. The authors don't just extol but explain exactly how to harness digital technology with great attention to detail and specifics. Throughout, you are signposted to research, evidence and existing implementation with some checklists for application and frequently asked questions (FAQs) answered too. All the necessary insights required to move from pilot to permanent programme, along with team development and management considerations, are covered. Some of the case studies that narrate the improved confidence and independence of both carers and those they care for are genuinely moving, and if you are a finance director, be prepared to be stirred by the associated cost savings too.

The unwritten hypothesis of this guide is that the culture of learned dependency has to end. We all have to become more intentional about our health and, for professionals, this means accepting and promoting the inherent dignity and right to information of those that we serve. Equipped with knowledge and understanding, people can become active 'participatients', depending less on professionals and thus using precious NHS resources more appropriately. It does require a changed dynamic and transitions are rarely smooth, but this journey is worth it.

It is an honour to be able to recommend this book, knowing both the passion and commitment that have driven the authors, and something of the resulting improvement in people's lived experiences. It deserves to be found in the hands of everyone who works in health and care, because patients need to reap the benefits of digital healthcare.

Julia Manning
BSc(Hons) MCOptom FRSA
Chief Executive 2020health
1st Floor Devon House,
171–177 Great Portland Street,
London W1W 5PQ
07973 312358 | www.2020health.org

2020health is an independent, social enterprise think tank working to improve health through research, campaigning, networking and relationships. We do not lobby on behalf of companies, organisations or individuals and retain editorial control of all our publications.

Preface

This book captures many good examples of technology enabled care services (TECS). The authors are innovative leaders who have made TECS happen in their setting or organisation for a range of applications and users, taken up at the 'front line'. They share their insights in how to engage patients or service users and practitioner users of TECS. They focus on 'how to do it' – not just about redesigning services and setting up the support structures, but about making delivery happen in virtual ways.

A main theme transmitted throughout the three parts of the book is the imperative to support care professionals in making the best use of technology and data (about a person's condition) through: enhanced competency and capability, leadership, professionalism and collaborative/cooperative working. Every chapter in this book gives colour to each of these skills and should enthuse readers to see how the knowledge and skills can be achieved – and by putting them into practice make a real difference.

The UK is regarded as one of the best places in the world to evolve, design, manufacture and adopt twenty-first-century healthcare and life sciences technologies, so it is just the right time to publish this book – and relay how to make that adoption and dissemination happen at the front line.

The focus of this book is on frontline innovation with new modes of delivery of healthcare, and this is inevitably a rapidly growing and changing area. Things are moving on all the time and we recommend readers become increasingly active in supporting personalisation of those for whom they provide care and activating integrated working between health and social care. We should highlight opportunities for improved awareness of existing and emerging technologies by the public, including greater emphasis on the potential to self purchase as these types of technologies become increasingly mainstream and available. As time goes by, the public are starting to realise that it is no longer viable to rely on the state (NHS and Local Authorities) for provision of every element of self care.

We have created a website associated with this book so that we can publish new information, other updates and additional material as it evolves – see http://bit.ly/digitalhealthupdate

Disclaimer

All the documents, ideas and suggestions included in the content of this book are intended to inform readers about others' experiences and approaches to the delivery of digital healthcare in health and social care settings. The content is not a substitute for national advice and guidance from professional or regulatory organisations. While every effort has been made to include accurate and up to date information about legal requirements, descriptors of IT infrastructure and other resources such as hyperlinked websites, knowledge and understanding are constantly evolving and being updated. So you need to use the content of the book to learn more about how you can adopt or enhance your use of digital healthcare and weigh up the choices, information and guidance for your own circumstances. Inclusion of named agencies, websites, companies, services or publications in this book does not constitute a recommendation or endorsement.

About the authors

Professor Ruth Chambers OBE

Ruth is an experienced GP, having worked for more than 30 years in different practices along with many lead roles in academia, the Royal College of General Practitioners, Department of Health, learning and development, and various clinical interests – all focused on disseminating best practice in healthcare. Ruth's main driver is her passion to improve the quality of patient care across the NHS; she has co-led an effective quality improvement scheme with underpinning learning and development in Stoke-on-Trent.

Ruth is always thinking of new ideas – and actually puts some into practice, testing out innovations in creative ways, then disseminating learning as widely as energy levels and opportunities allow. Currently that is as clinical Chair of Stoke-on-Trent Clinical Commissioning Group (CCG) and clinical lead for the West Midlands Academic Health Science Network (WMAHSN)-funded programme to promote person-centred care exemplars of technology enabled care services (TECS).

Specific lifetime achievements: Ruth has written 69 books as main or co-author; three for the general public, the rest for healthcare staff. Some have been translated into Japanese, Italian and Korean. Many of these books have been used in university/NHS courses across the UK and abroad. Those for the general public (on heart disease, back pain and stress) have had good reviews and sales.

Ruth.Chambers@stoke.nhs.uk

Jayne Birch-Jones

Having a master's in health service research, Jayne has spent much of her 32-year NHS career working as a nurse, health informatics professional and most recently as an independent programme manager.

Jayne was instrumental in identifying the potential of simple telehealth (STH) as being able to realise significant 'invest to save' benefits, establishing it as a programme of work and implementing it across the whole of Nottinghamshire's health and social care community, where it is now a mainstreamed operationalised service. Jayne also provided operational support to the national AIM (Advice and Interactive Messaging) for Health programme, advising other organisations on how to implement Florence (Flo) simple telehealth.

Jayne has authored and co-authored several published articles describing her experiences of implementation and evaluation of telehealth.

Currently Jayne is working as a TECS programme consultant with the East Midlands Academic Health Science Network (EMAHSN), developing a TECS programme.

Marc Schmid

Marc has had a career spanning over 20 years in media and communications. Having worked as a PR advisor to a member of the European Parliament and member of Parliament, he has developed a career at a senior level working across communications in local government and the NHS.

He is the communications and digital lead for the Pennine Lancashire Health Transformation Board and a member of the Lancashire Digital Board. He is also seconded to the Lancashire Care Foundation Trust to support the digital health Lancashire programme with particular responsibility for connecting communities through digital means. In these roles, and as a director of a social enterprise, Redmoor Communications, he has delivered digital projects across education, the NHS and local government for the last eight years as well as part of an apprentice training programme he delivered for the Department for Work and Pensions (DWP). With most of his attention focused on the health portfolio, Marc has worked across the West Midlands and North West England developing the use of social media in primary and secondary care as well as training and developing health and social care staff to use digital modes of delivery as part of the transformation agenda.

As part of these projects he is developing peer to peer support networks among patients linked to GP practices or hospitals. He has also been developing the use of Skype technology for use in primary care and with hospitals where interpreters are required for patient care.

Marc also delivers innovative health journalism projects in schools for public health where pupils are given research and writing tasks on a host of public health subjects such as smoking, road safety, diet and alcohol.

In his spare time Marc is a qualified rugby league and rugby union coach and coaches children aged between 8 and 11 years for Leyland Warriors RLFC and Wigan RUFC.

Twitter @marcschmid

Jim Ellam

Jim originally trained as a social worker and has worked within a wide variety of residential, hospital and community social care teams in London, Worcestershire and, since 2000, in Staffordshire.

Since 2008 Jim has worked in commissioning, leading on assistive technology, supporting service transformation and personalised care. Jim works closely with partner agencies to encourage the utilisation of the full range of technology solutions from simple to complex types and he is committed to supporting people to live independently, exercising choice and control over their lives, and supporting those who provide care.

Dr Lizzie Cottrell

Lizzie is a clinical lecturer at Keele University, spending half her working life as a salaried GP and the other half specialising in evaluation and research relating to health service provision. Lizzie has recently completed her PhD which has been focused on investigating attitudes, beliefs and behaviours of GPs regarding the management of chronic knee pain. This has led to an interest in trying to better understand the behaviours of GPs. Lizzie has written books for medical students and medical educators. Throughout her GP training and since qualification, Lizzie has evaluated a local health service quality improvement scheme and local and national STH initiatives; the findings have been disseminated at national conferences and in peer-reviewed journals.

Lizzie likes to combine her academic and clinical experience to promote better practice in her local clinical environment and more widely. For example, she has published two good-quality audits in peer-reviewed journals about gout and inflammatory arthritis and has most recently published a clinical intelligence article about Addison's disease in the *British Journal of General Practice*. Lizzie is a peer-reviewer for many health journals and has recently commenced a post as an editorial board member for the 'Knowledge, attitudes, behaviours, education and communication' section of *BMC Family Practice*.

Richard Haynes

Richard has a vast amount of knowledge and experience across the care spectrum, working for local and central government. For example, he has previously delivered modernised day care services, specialist dementia services, home care reablement, electronic home care call monitoring, provided residential care, personalised budgets and implemented the retail model for community equipment. His knowledge of telecare, telehealth and assistive technology (AT) services is second to none. Richard has won two national awards for work in the public sector, from the *Local Government Association* and *Municipal Journal*, related to social work, and one for innovative service delivery of AT.

Richard has worked with the Department of Health and Department of Work and Pensions. He is a certified PRINCE2 practitioner and has trained in other related tools including Managing Successful Programmes and Management of Risk.

Richard is the founding director of The Community Gateway CIC, a social enterprise with a genuine and passionate interest in communities and people: *see* ww.communitygateway.co.uk/

Lisa Taylor

Lisa is a specialist and thought leader in the development of the STH Florence methodology. She enjoys supporting positive change to deliver improvements in quality outcomes for patients and their families. Lisa has worked within the NHS for over 15 years, across primary care, acute and community services in operational and multi-agency redesign roles at local, regional and national levels. Lisa has a BA(Hons) in economics and an MBA and also plays a leading inspirational role in the ongoing international NHS England/US Department of Veterans Affairs (NHSE/VA) exchange programme.

Lisa specialises in the use of innovative personalised models of care delivery to achieve better and faster outcomes where patient and clinician feel involved, equipped and enabled. Lisa has a keen focus on evaluation and dissemination of best practice, with recent research focusing on the barriers and enablers to STH's adoption and diffusion. Having been closely involved with Florence's early implementation and infrastructure, Lisa now uses this experience to enable organisations across the UK to develop and improve their capability and maturity with the STH methodology and to share best practice.

John Uttley

After graduating with a master's degree in European and international law, John joined the NHS in an IT role. He has 18 years' experience in the NHS (acute and primary care), mostly in senior management and director roles (including as chief information officer). He is currently involved in the evolution of one of the most successful Commissioning Support Units (CSUs) in England, from its inception as the e-Innovations director. Midlands and Lancashire CSU's e-Innovations department has a dedicated team of experts who represent the CSU's commitment to fund innovation, which will drive benefits for patients and Clinical Commissioning Groups (CCGs) and other NHS trust customers.

John has pioneered the creation of the UK's first real-time urgent care tracker, which enables operational and medical teams to better manage the flow of patients within the urgent care system. The team led by John has also created a case management tool based on evidence from research, which has resulted in a *BMJ* open publication on the *benefits of joining datasets to identify cohorts of patients,* resulting in improved patient outcomes.

John is also leading on England's largest primary care Virtual Desktop Infrastructure (VDI) project for Birmingham Cross City CCG. This technology will revolutionise the way in which the CCG provides IT services to GPs, and will, more importantly, improve patient care, increase clinicians' productivity and reduce costs.

John has significant experience in telehealth, including working on an international project with the US Department of Veterans Affairs to create a telehealth application. At present John is working with a small number of truly innovative telehealth solutions providers, with pilots planned with a number of CCG and trust customers.

John has close ties with Keele University's Health Service Research Unit, and is an honorary research fellow with the Institute of Science Technology and Medicine (iSTM). He is working with both the West Midlands and Greater

Manchester Academic Health Science Networks on various projects, which aim to drive innovation and create a digital economy in our health system.

Ciaron Hoye

Ciaron Hoye is the senior information officer at NHS Birmingham Cross City CCG, the fourth largest CCG in the country, and is the digital lead for the wider Birmingham digital economy, including primary and secondary care organisations covering a population of 1.8 million patients. He has a strong track record of bringing digital innovation into the NHS, with a particular focus on leveraging technology and machine learning to help service clinician and patient needs.

Part One

What is digital healthcare?

Chapter 1

Where we are now with technology enabled care and services

Dr Ruth Chambers

Digital technology offers great opportunities for transforming health and social care services and associated outcomes, and for improving the experiences of patients or service users and their carers.

Despite the common usage of the Internet and other technologies in people's personal lives, take up of telehealth and technology enabled delivery of care across the NHS and social care settings has been very slow. There are many national strategies that promote the potential benefits to be gained from integrating technology into the wide-scale delivery of care – in particular Skype, telecare and telehealth. There has also been much discussion about how to minimise the barriers to its deployment by NHS and social care organisations, health and social care practitioners and managers, and patients or service users and their carers in the move to enhance high-quality, financially sustainable care in the future.[1–5]

There is a national drive to focus on 'supporting people in making the right health and care choices through digital access to health and care information and transactions'.[2,4] This should result in enhanced prevention and self-care and improved quality of delivery of care as well as contribute to future sustainability of health and social care services. The five 'big enablers' of the shift in modernising healthcare are thought to be: finance, integration, workforce, technology and empowerment.[6] Technology enabled care services (TECS) can therefore underpin more effective and productive working and thus save money, aid integration across health and social care settings, support the workforce in more efficient and virtual delivery of care as well as empower citizens.

The infrastructure needed to make TECS work effectively as integrated care includes ready access to digital patient records by health and social care professionals – in a paperless culture. People's real-time health and social care records need to be shared according to national technical and professional data standards within and across care settings. Practitioners can then share information along patient pathways with informed consent, governance and assurance of safeguards.[4] This extended sharing of a person's care records will include interactions with individual citizens too.

If we focus technology enabled care on all the common organisational priorities in health and social care settings we will be able to show that successful remote delivery of care:

- saves money (e.g. fewer unplanned hospital admissions, less medication wastage)
- is more convenient (for patients, carers and practitioners)
- enhances productivity of NHS or social care teams (e.g. fewer home visits or face-to-face consultations)
- enhances clinical outcomes (so people live longer in a healthier state).

But it takes time – and many new technology enabled care schemes can take up to three years to set up, recruit or train the workforce and achieve impact from delivery of the scheme.[7]

We do need to optimise the power of individuals to take more responsibility for self-care and shared management of their conditions and their lifestyle habits, hopefully aiding prevention and management of any long-term illnesses. This might be via personalised care plans, with technologies being an option to help people track and analyse their own health data, and social innovation with different approaches to peer support, such as via social media.[8] We should make best use of the Internet access that nearly 90% of UK adults have.[9]

The vision for TECS for all NHS organisations and local authorities in the UK is to optimise the 'potential of technology to transform traditional models of care and support and to enable greater self-management of care and support people and their carers to be as independent as possible'.[10] This will empower people of all ages to take greater responsibility for their own health and well-being and make their own choices, with more control over their own health and lives. It will also reduce admissions and readmissions to hospital and enhance long-term care of older people. The goal is also to find particular technology and TECS that work in trusted ways for the clinical team or individual practitioner using them.

NHS England promotes the incorporation of TECS in all commissioning and organisational delivery of care plans. The range of TECS includes: telehealth, telecare, telemedicine, Skype or video consultations and apps;[11] but social media channels of communication should be included too.

The national vision for TECS is that everyone with a long-term condition should be routinely reviewed as to what technology might be appropriate to help them or their carers, as well as health and social care professionals, to better manage their conditions or lifestyle habits. Effective technology should therefore enable appropriate planned interventions for patients with greatest need, to improve the quality and timeliness of the delivery of their care.

With people living longer and the proportion of older people in our society growing, pressure is placed on current and future health and social care resources. More proactive prevention is necessary for all individuals with chronic health conditions or adverse lifestyle habits. TECS can improve access to care and provide prompt responses for the older population, hopefully allowing earlier intervention. With these challenges comes high demand on services, requiring new and innovative approaches to delivering care.

Given the significant shortage of financial and clinical resources, better use of TECS may mean that the gap between health needs and available resources is not as wide as anticipated. Doctors and other clinicians will never be replaced as direct providers of acute healthcare (unless by robots?), but what we can do is to utilise TECS to address public health and self-care aspects of care, in order to free up clinician time for seriously ill patients.

While all this progress and transformation of care is exciting, we need to continue to protect personal data and ensure that usage and access is in line with information governance requirements, in order to assure patients of the confidentiality of their personal information.

Collaborative working via TECS

TECS are a combination of equipment, information, monitoring and response that can help clinicians and patients to manage a person's health and social care. There might be a particular focus on managing long-term conditions (LTCs) effectively, so preventing avoidable deterioration or minimising the consequences of the conditions. This might be through titration of medication, reminders to take medication regularly or attend review appointments, relaying of bodily symptoms, signs or measures by remote means, encouraging improved lifestyle habits, or giving patients (and clinicians) more understanding of their conditions. The essential ingredient to the success of TECS is the dual management plan agreed between patient and clinician – with hopefully more than one clinician involved along the relevant patient pathway – interfacing between general practice, secondary care, mental health and community settings. It should be the drive to improve clinical outcomes for individual patients that dictates whether digital delivery is useful and, if so, what types of remote delivery of care suit the patient's needs and preferences for the resources available.

The role of a practitioner or manager will be to spot, adopt and roll out technological solutions and enhancements for cost-effective delivery of safe, good-quality care for people with LTCs in their patient population. The role is also to prioritise anticipatory care focused on local priorities so as to minimise avoidable healthcare usage.

> Keele University and Stoke-on-Trent Clinical Commissioning Group (CCG) have developed a really useful website: www.digitalhealthsot.nhs.uk. This online resource for clinicians, commissioners and patients describes all types of technology enabled care and has been developed to cover a wide range of TECS initiatives. These include informational videos about LTCs and 'how to do it' about technology that can support patients, such as video conferencing for patient consultation.

Virtual access to patient records

With the required infrastructure requirements being addressed nationally, the potential for TECS use is endless. The future is fast approaching and technologies are constantly evolving, adapting and improving around us. The Industrial Revolution lasted for 80 years. The digital revolution started in 1980 and if it lasts as long as its industrial predecessor, it has another 44 years to go! The health-related digital revolution only started recently and is therefore just in its infancy, with many years of advancement ahead of it.

There is a UK-wide push to publish data on individual teams' and practitioners' everyday practice, and to continuously invite individual patients' feedback – comments, complaints and suggestions. Online access in general practice to a person's medical records, booking of appointments and ordering repeat prescriptions is usually available. Individuals can (or will be able to, in some cases) request that access to their records is extended to other clinicians; or the person use an appropriate app to link to their medical record of their clinical condition and its clinical management. All this improved access to a person's medical records must be underpinned by appropriate clinical governance for safe care management and information governance for conserving patient confidentiality and safe data sharing. Recent legislation has endorsed the use of a person's

NHS number so that all organisations in health and social care can identify the individual person in the same way with a view to sharing personal data in valid, reliable and safe ways.[12]

Patient online access

People are increasingly choosing to book appointments at their general practice and order repeat prescriptions online. Some want to view their own health records online. They are used to the out of working hours system for accessing medical advice or proceeding to a consultation after telephone triage. Soon, hopefully, people in England will be able to view their GP records, including blood test results, appointment records and medical histories, and speak to their doctor online or by a video link, via their smartphones or apps. There should be associated benefits from such information sharing including increased patient safety with fewer mistakes, duplications or erroneous drug doses; hopefully fewer unnecessary phone calls to practices if patients can book or cancel their appointments; and increased ability for patients to make informed decisions about their health and well-being.[13] But there are potential risks too: people might be coerced by family members or friends to share access to their medical records with potential harm and safeguarding issues if there is sensitive information in the content. If online services become the prime way to book appointments, those who are more technologically able might snap up the majority of appointments at the expense of poorer people who live without home Internet access or are not digitally competent.

Some ambulance services share patient records through digital systems with accident and emergency teams; some healthcare providers interact with others in different settings through shared records or multidisciplinary interactions via a Skype 'meeting' with or without the patient present in person.

How can virtual access to care help the general public?

The adoption of digital technology is happening all around us. People are increasingly using digital communications in their everyday lives, whether that be online shopping, Internet banking, Skype or FaceTime calls with relatives and friends or using apps to search for information or services. Over-55 year olds appear to be the fastest growing age group in terms of Internet usage. These technologies will support self-care, support carers and help people better manage their LTCs.

For patients: flexible access, including access to video, Skype consultations and social media, can lead to:

- better access to health services
- care closer to home
- automated interaction with general practice-based clinician by patient (and carer)

- better time management for carers
- greater flexibility in how patients access healthcare.

More productive delivery of digital care might provide:

- teleconsultation integrated into care pathways with technology enabled services in practice and care/nursing home settings
- fewer unnecessary face-to-face consultations for follow-up care of LTCs or redressing adverse lifestyle habits
- better time management
- learning by doing and sharing care; being more confident and competent with Skype or video consultations
- reduced healthcare usage, e.g. unplanned hospital admissions, use of A&E, face-to-face consultations with patient/clinician
- multidisciplinary team virtual meetings
- reduced health inequalities as those whose work or care responsibilities make daytime access difficult have improved access to care
- a behaviour change in patients with rapid anticipatory care that improves self-care and compliance with medication/interventions, and prevents deterioration of health conditions
- enhanced patient quality of life, while living with their LTCs
- regular follow-up care with appropriate healthcare staff
- better integration between community and acute care settings, to ensure that patients are not admitted inappropriately and can remain within their residential setting
- reassurance and support to care home staff
- earlier discharge from hospital.

The use of technology, such as vital signs monitoring and communication with patients through the use of telehealth equipment, should enable more effective management of resources, as it frees clinicians to focus on and engage in treating and reviewing a housebound patient's medical condition, rather than spending time travelling to the patient's home or care home.

The added advantages of technology from a patient's perspective are their increased ability and confidence to self-manage their health conditions. Interactive communication and information that has a focused purpose may well increase their adherence to clinical interventions and improve lifestyle behaviour. Such change in behaviour (physical and psychological) is likely to continue after the digital mode of delivery is withdrawn (e.g. they might continue ongoing home monitoring of blood pressure) once the patient is empowered and understands the significance of their condition and agreed shared care. This improved virtual access to health or social care is a great help if they have commitments that limit usual access arrangements; for example, because they are carers, work shifts or are away from their home base.

Choice of technology

Choosing the type of technology for digital delivery of care will depend on what is available locally, or is affordable within financial and other resource constraints, maybe after a risk/benefit analysis to match the strategy and local or national priorities. It will also depend on the needs and preferences of a particular patient or service user, their capability (e.g. cognitive function or familiarity with a type of technology or willingness to learn or interact) and the competence of their health or social care professionals or carers. A friend or family member might be prepared to help them out in the use of a particular technology and extend the choice of what is affordable or available.

Choice of technology to underpin the clinical or social interventions will also depend on what support services are available. So, for example, where the functioning of the technology is interactive and the patient's or service user's responses are rated on a scale ranging from 'good' or 'no problems' to 'concerns' or 'red alert', there will need to be a health or social care response service. This might be simple and cheap, such as automated response messaging that guides and signposts the user to the next steps they should take (what/who/how/when) or provides a real-time or timed active response from a clinician or carer (by text or voice via telephone or face to face depending on purpose or pre-agreed protocol). The patient or service user must have given informed consent to the nature of this interaction and extent of support available and there should be written proof that they consented to an automated interaction, if that is the case.

All of these aspects should have been considered at a pan-organisational level where patient safety and mitigation of risks are covered in a 'privacy impact assessment', the 'standard operating procedure', 'information governance' and 'clinical governance' documents approved by the respective Caldicott Guardian. It may be that there is a commissioning board, or health and well-being board, to sign off such policies and aid synchronisation across local NHS, local authority, and third sector or voluntary group settings. This promotes multi-provider delivery and integrated care.

Range of technology commonly used in health and social care settings

Telemedicine

'Telemedicine' is a term that has varied interpretations. It sometimes relates to the use of sensors and electronic means of communication from one clinician to another, to aid diagnosis and clinical management; this might typically be by a pre-booked video conference between GP or community nurse and consultant for a shared patient consultation (the patient may or may not be present too).[11] Sometimes the term 'telemedicine' has a wider application, such as 'distance medicine using information and communication technologies to examine, monitor, treat and care for patients over a distance ... both within and between all kinds of healthcare institutions as well as to monitor and provide support to patients living at home'.[11] Even a consultation generated by a clinician phoning an individual patient to relay information might be considered as telemedicine by some.

There is much debate as to the benefits and challenges of telemedicine. On the positive side, video consultation should be more convenient for patients and potentially save costs of travel (for health and social care staff and patients/ service users); on the negative side, there are significant technical, logistical and regulatory challenges and potential clinical risks.[14] Read more about telemedicine in Chapter 5.

Skype

Skype or video consultation can provide a remote facility for clinicians to deliver face-to-face care without the patient attending an in-person consultation. It doesn't directly replace face-to-face meetings but can be used in an integral way for the right person as an alternative to the patient attending a clinic session or the clinician making a home visit.

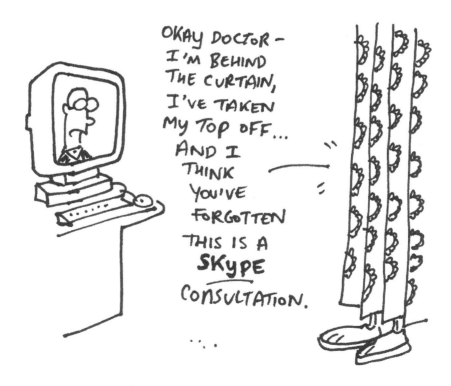

Video consultation might be provided via an encrypted connection rather than a non-confidential video interaction via Skype. Skype might be set up between the clinician and a patient who has their own access to Skype via their mobile phone, tablet, computer or other device; or it might be set up for clinician to clinician interaction for a remote peer professional meeting or between practitioners in different settings (such as acute hospital and general practice settings). Sometimes connectivity can be difficult, such as in multi-dwelling occupancies such as a care home with flats for independent residents, or with particular mobile phone services. This type of delivery of care has become increasingly well established in rural communities where travel can be challenging, such as remote areas in Australia. People with disabilities or who have mobility issues or mental health problems such as agoraphobia can really welcome video conferencing or Skype which enhances access and availability of care. According to Greenhalgh *et al.*, 'Having a multidisciplinary team working on a Skype consultation or video or teleconference with team, carer and patient stops people having to go in for an appointment and saves money.'[15]

Read more about teleconsultation in Chapter 5.

Telecare

Telecare or assistive technology (AT) maintains or improves the well-being and independence of people with cognitive, physical or communication difficulties. This might include jar openers, bath seats or stairlifts, and electronic sensors and aids that make a home environment safer or which may link to a triage system where alerts can be relayed to social or healthcare teams.[11,16] When a telephone network is included, the AT might be termed 'telecare', in which the monitoring of care relates to personal safety, security and home environmental risks via communication over a distance by telephone (mobile phone or landline). Sometimes a non-clinical triage centre is established to monitor users' responses in real time and trigger face-to-face or other direct help if agreed thresholds are breached – as in Example 1.1. In other systems the monitoring might be automated and overseen intermittently. Telecare also includes the use of electronic sensors and aids to make the home environment safer so that people are more secure and live independently.

It may be that some people prefer face-to-face personal delivery of care from, for example, community nurses or social care workers with whom they've developed good relationships. They might resent substitution of technology as an alternative method of delivery, as this might make them feel more isolated. Although some people prefer personal face-to-face delivery that reduces their social isolation, their practitioner or local service pathways might need to prioritise a more effective and productive type of TECS that supplements or replaces face-to-face health or social care.

There is a relatively low uptake of telecare or AT by older people. One way forward for potential users and their carers is to co-design future technology applications and services, evolving ways to co-produce useful and useable solutions.[17]

Read more about telecare and AT in Chapters 3 and 4.

EXAMPLE 1.1 Stoke-on-Trent City Council Telecare Service

The telecare service provides expertise and technology for remote monitoring of clients at home or in residential settings.

Provision of telecare services includes the assessment, provision and monitoring of sensors in the person's home. When the sensors are activated they communicate automatically with the 24/7 control centre where staff can talk to the person to find out the problem, and dispatch a suitable response when and where required. These sensors include:

- community alarm pendant worn by the person
- smoke alarm
- bed occupancy sensor (pressure pad) to detect if a person has left their bed, or not returned to bed
- chair occupancy sensor
- door contacts (e.g. to convey an alert about a wandering client)
- passive sensors (to detect movement or absence of movement)
- fall detectors
- automated pill dispenser
- flood detector (for overflowing bath, sink etc.)
- carbon monoxide detector (to detect a faulty fire/heater)
- temperature extremes sensor (to show if a house is getting too hot or cold)
- epilepsy sensor (based on detecting the vibration and noise of different types of seizure)
- enuresis sensor
- combinations of such sensors in a 'just checking' system which can be used to assess a person's activity and mobility at home over a defined time period.

Telehealth

Telehealth includes linked equipment, monitoring and responses that can help individual people to remain independent at home.[11] So a telehealth deployment might relay specific physiological data from patients at work or in their homes to clinicians in a health setting to support informed (and hopefully shared) decisions about their clinical management. Telehealth might underpin a 'virtual ward' of specific patients with remote monitoring of their vital signs that is overseen by specific clinicians. Telehealth can relay a patient's vital signs or test results or bodily measures to clinicians caring for them from afar – in real time or close to real time. A great advantage is that patients or service users (and their carers) are much more aware of how their body is functioning and whether their condition is controlled (or not!).

The international code of practice for telehealth services[16] includes sections on:

- ethical perspectives
- governance and financial issues
- personal information management
- staff management
- contact with users and carers
- interpretation of responses to information
- communications networks
- hardware and technological considerations.

The code of practice domains[16] cover:

- health/motivational coaching and advice
- activity and lifestyle monitoring
- safeguarding and monitoring in care settings
- gait, seizure and falls prediction and management
- point of care testing and diagnoses
- vital signs monitoring
- mobile health technology systems
- medication or therapy adherence
- rehabilitation and (re)ablement
- responses to adverse events and incidents
- teleconsultations and virtual presence.

Read more about telehealth in Chapter 2.

Apps

Around three-quarters of adults in the UK have a smartphone.[18] Already smartphones are being used for medical applications, coupled with wearable biosensors, and are able to sense, analyse and display vital signs, and generate alerts to significant changes or deterioration, highlighting escalation of a condition which can then be identified and addressed in a timely and proactive way. As part of this smartphone revolution, attachments that can track heart rhythms or monitor mental health via apps can lead to better health outcomes while being more convenient for the patient, their carer and their clinicians.

Health-related apps are often bought or obtained by individual members of the public and uploaded onto their mobile phone or tablet or accessed via website – as in Example 1.2. Health apps can enhance a person's understanding of their health condition and empower them to manage their health or to be more aware of their lifestyle habits and the associated effects on them. An app might support delivery of health or social care, maybe enabling sharing of provision of care across care settings. Uses of a health app include:

- enabling remote monitoring of a patient's adherence to an intervention or medication, or bodily measurements such as their weight

- supporting self-diagnosis or monitoring
- providing professional support and education
- signposting to appropriate services
- sharing visual images and information to enable remote diagnosis
- underpinning clinical networks.

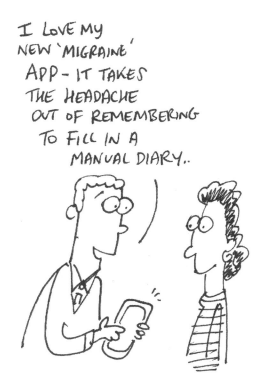

EXAMPLE 1.2   Migraine diary app

See http://apps.nhs.uk/app/migraine-diary/
This app provides a diary for people with migraine. The diary content is derived from Patient.co.uk. The diary lets the user track their symptoms, log possible triggers, record medication taken and access information about migraine and possible interventions and treatment.

The app is freely available. The user can capture:

- severity of the pain
- length of migraine attack
- whether there was an aura
- nausea or sickness
- possible triggers
- medication taken.

Users are advised that recorded details of their migraine attacks can help:

- their doctor make a firm diagnosis of migraine
- them recognise warning signs of an attack
- them identify triggers
- them assess whether their treatment is working.

The NHS in England has an online apps library: http://apps.nhs.uk/ (currently being updated). Apps that are loaded in this library are regarded as being 'clinically safe'. There are European regulations about medical apps; a 'CE' mark confirms that an app has been deemed to meet essential criteria, works and is clinically safe. Apps that are for administrative functions, or give general guidance or support training, are not classed as 'medical' and thus do not require accreditation. Those that provide personalised advice and are diagnostic or used for medical purposes such as calculation of treatment are regarded as 'medical' apps and thus do need a 'CE' mark.

Read more about apps in Chapter 6.

Social media

There are various ways in which social media can support health and social care organisations or teams. It can work with health communities, motivating them and linking with services offered by the NHS or social care. Social media can also support the introduction of technology, empowering patients or service users to take personal responsibility for their health by giving them access to information, so reducing the need for face-to-face consultation. Social media can also motivate people who may be experiencing significant life changes, bringing them into contact with people suffering from similar conditions. Often these support networks are via closed groups and forums.

Read more about social media in Chapter 7 or access the social media toolkit on www.digitalhealthsot.nhs.uk

Telephone consultations

There's a lot of emphasis on the types of technology that can be used for digital delivery of care – especially mobile phones and tablets. The benefits to patients or service users come from the enhanced delivery of clinical or social care and associated shared care management, not from a particular type of digital mode of delivery.

Telephone consultations (via landline or mobile phone) have been in place for decades between care practitioner and patient. Sometimes that is because the patient prefers a phone consultation for convenience; for example, they do not need to take time off work to attend or leave the person they are caring for. Sometimes a clinician might initiate it because they want to feed back test results and discuss the next steps, or modify a treatment or intervention as a stepped management plan; or a GP might initiate a phone call after communication from other care providers such as a hospital consultant or community nurse.

There are information governance and clinical governance issues relating to telephone consultations, including confidentiality, documentation and safety netting. The clinician initiating the call will need to be sure that they are talking to the 'patient' whose symptoms, treatments or records they are discussing. The clinician will need to practise safe, comprehensive history taking if they are making a diagnosis or altering treatment. They will need to take care to make appropriate levels of decision by phone, when they cannot see the patient, or take bodily measurements. If they are relying on a patient's reported measurement, they will need to be sure that the equipment and way it is used is reliable and valid.

Telephone triage can work well, such as for patients seeking a consultation with, or home visit by, a GP, or for an out-of-hours service. Patients in most need can be prioritised and others fitted around, while patients who would otherwise have had to take time off work to attend the GP's surgery can be safely advised or treated remotely via the phone consultation. Those clinicians doing the telephone triage during working hours need a brief with some basic information about the patient's current condition (symptoms) or queries, along with other knowledge from the patient's records to be able to prioritise which patients to phone back and which to see face to face or refer on elsewhere as soon as possible.

Email healthcare services

The secure email standard is available at: http://systems.hscic.gov.uk/nhsmail/future/service/security/index_html. This includes guidance on policies and procedures relating to NHSmail – for those with or without an N3 NHS connection. The email standard has been developed to support the secure exchange of sensitive information between health and social care organisations using secure email services – as utilised in Example 1.3.

If a clinician or carer is emailing a patient or service user, they will need to remember that this interaction will not be via a secure encrypted exchange; others might read the recipient's email sent by their clinician or carer if left about or if an incorrect email address is used.

EXAMPLE 1.3   Secure email pilot to replace faxing by care homes

A secure email pilot project has been completed in Shropshire Care Homes, whereby staff emailed patient information securely and rapidly. This pilot has defined the benefits of secure email across healthcare and local authority boundaries in readiness for the national rollout to all social care organisations.[19]

In Denmark, email consultation is a mandatory element of general practice provision, with the email consultation being directly incorporated into the patient's electronic record.

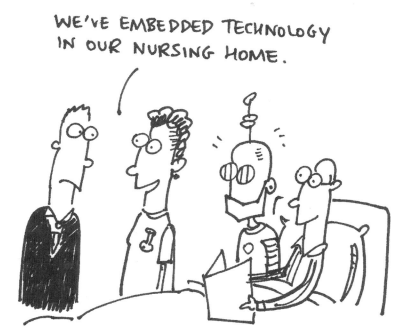

Selecting the right type of TECS

Selecting the right type of TECS for a particular person, or pathway, should result in:

- improved patient empowerment, e.g. self-management, agreed titration of medication etc. to achieve improved clinical outcomes
- fewer avoidable hospital (re)admissions and visits to A&E, saving NHS or social care resources
- promotion of good patient lifestyles, e.g. managing obesity, smoking cessation, tackling alcohol misuse, thus enhancing quality of life and prolonging life expectancy
- enhanced shared clinician or patient management of long-term conditions, such as chronic obstructive pulmonary disease (COPD), asthma, diabetes, heart failure and hypertension as well as other health problems like dementia, thus preventing deterioration of those chronic health conditions
- consistent application of best practice in clinical management along patient pathways spanning all health settings: general practice, pharmacy, community care and acute and mental healthcare
- extended availability and accessibility of patients to a variety of technologies: including interactive webcams/Skype, video links, mobile

phone texting, fixed or wireless communication via smartphones and tablets, health apps and telephone consulting

- enhanced competence and expertise in digital delivery and experience in applying telehealth – as individual health or social care professionals or teams for a range of TECS in local, national and international settings.

At present, the offer of telehealth, telecare (AT) or video consultation seems ad hoc in any health or social care setting and depends on the clinician's or carer's enthusiasm for technology enabled care, their awareness, competence and capability, or the availability of a range of technology equipment or support.

Individuals with an LTC (or at risk of developing one) should be offered a TECS assessment – with the clinician or social worker completing a checklist. This TECS assessment process should take a holistic view of an individual's health and social care needs and suitability for technology enabled care, with the aim of giving the patient as much control and participation as they want in the management of their condition or in redressing adverse lifestyle habits.

TECS should be a key element of any global healthcare strategy that addresses the need for any country to provide cost-effective care for its ageing population and the increasing numbers with LTCs.

Overcoming the challenges to integration of TECS[20,21]

Strategies and linked implementation plans for TECS must be focused on service developments and improvements that are (likely to be) cost effective and which solve current challenges such as capacity issues facing general practice. In order to be successful, redesigned services should be relatively easy to deliver and appeal to patients.

To take TECS forward at pace we need to:

1. establish and support leaders and champions of TECS throughout the commissioning cycle to communicate the benefits and drive change – from envisaging and consultation stages, to procurement and defining service specifications, training and rollout, delivery and ongoing evaluation
2. enable patient and public involvement and engagement; patients could co-drive digital delivery of care
3. use telehealth or other digital modes of delivery such as Skype, telecare (AT), teleconsultations or telediagnostics to drive person-centred, integrated care rather than standalone solutions
4. focus digital delivery of care on areas in patient pathways where enhancing self-care has a substantial impact by improving patients' clinical outcomes and/or reducing avoidable healthcare usage
5. anticipate consequence costs, such as increased frequency of clinician alerts
6. train health and social care professionals: enhance workforce competencies and capabilities for the rollout of technology enabled care

7. match the mode of digital delivery of care to suit the patient population – selected mode or individualised for their needs and preferences, helping to overcome barriers to accessing healthcare for some marginalised groups[22]

8. rigorously evaluate any implementation or trial of TECS; such information will underpin any future business cases

9. utilise improvement tools to underpin commissioning and service improvement – leadership, transformational change and service redesign

10. work closely with all stakeholders to integrate technology in care to improve outcomes for all services; redress ongoing issues in constructive ways before progress with rollout is stalled.

Information sources to help you to select or provide the right TECS for your purpose

- Telecare Services Association: to see some widely used telecare and telehealth services: www.telecare.org.uk/consumer-services/telecare-and-telehealth

- www.mickshouse.info: this website shows telecare sensors and explains their functionality.

- www.independentforlonger.com/

- Disabled Living Foundation (DLF), the 'Personal alarm systems and telecare factsheet' provides information on types of telecare systems for specific difficulties; see: www.dlf.org.uk/factsheets/telecare?gclid=CjwKEAj w68ufBRDt0Zmrn4W_8AwSJADcjp1cr4G14MSXdNQZg2q5c6P_VLw NJLf63coWVYGS4srgdhoCDXnw_wcB

- 'AT Dementia' for technologies that support people with dementia and their carers: www.atdementia.org.uk/

- The HF Trust's virtual Smart House for technologies that people with learning disability may use at home to improve their independence and increase their safety: www.hftsmarthouse.org.uk/

- The King's Fund 'Information technologies' relays a view of the emerging app market: www.kingsfund.org.uk/time-to-think-differently/trends/ information-technologies/new-ways-using-digital-technologies

- www.orcha.co.uk: this website provides a platform of validated apps for professionals, patients and the public.

- http://everyday-life.co.uk: a decision support aid endorsed by West Midlands Academic Health Science Network designed to help patients and healthcare professionals to find the right technology solutions based on need, then connect them to a commercial company that can supply the technology.

- Royal College of Nursing, 'Telehealth and telecare': definitions, potential benefits and impact, and developments across the UK: www2.rcn.org.uk/ development/practice/e-health/telehealth_and_telecare

- www.nhs.uk is the domain hosting NHS Choices which provides a range of medical advice and healthcare information that is being developed as a clinically profiled directory of services encompassing health and social care services, and which will act as a 'digital hub' for services and be regarded as the 'digital front door' for online health services.

FAQs

Q1. So what type of digital technology would you recommend that my integrated locality care team start with?

A. Start with what the problem or issue is; don't be dominated by what technology is available. It's more about what outcomes you are trying to achieve for individuals receiving health or social care. The most important aspect of any digital mode of delivery of care is the shared care management plan that is agreed with the patient or service user before the technology is set up, or varied as the condition progresses and responds to the associated interventions. So consider the purpose of the aspects of care your team is delivering and the nature of the people who you are caring for, read up on what similar teams have done and achieved, and then draw up your delivery plan and business case for the types of technology that fit the scope and purpose you envisage.

Q2. Would you draw a line in supplying technology to certain age groups – maybe only focus on under-80 year olds?

A. Don't stereotype or discriminate against patient groups by excluding particular people from an offer of TECS. It is common for health or social care practitioners to assume that 'older' people will not be able to operate technology or be dependable in responding to interactive communication or feeding in bodily measurements. Much research and service evaluation and innumerable anecdotes show that many older people are very willing to engage in digital delivery of their care or involve a family member or other informal carer in aiding them in operating the allocated technology.

But we do need to plan for how we can upskill citizens to use health-related technology most appropriately or effectively; for example, to train people to use new systems and devices; and maybe creating a new workforce role of clinical technology specialist.[23]

References

1. NHS England (NHSE). *Five Year Forward View.* London: NHSE; 2014. Available at: www.england.nhs.uk/wp-content/uploads/2014/10/5yfv-web.pdf
2. NHS National Information Board. *Personalised Health and Care 2020: using data and technology to transform outcomes for patients and citizens; a framework for action.* London:

HM Government; 2014. Available at: www.gov.uk/government/uploads/system/uploads/attachment_data/file/384650/NIB_Report.pdf

3. Local Government Association. *Guide to the Care Act 2014 and the Implications for Providers*. London: Local Government Association; 2014. Available at: www.local.gov.uk

4. NHS National Information Board. *National Information Board's Workstream Roadmaps*. London: National Information Board; 2015. Available at: www.gov.uk/government/publications/national-information-boards-workstream-roadmaps

5. Elsy S, Rogan A. *Keeping the NHS Great: delivering technology enabled care services*. Sedlescombe: Good Governance Institute; 2014. Available at: www.good-governance.org.uk

6. Muir R, Quilter-Pinner H. *Powerful People: reinforcing the power of citizens and communities in health and care*. London: Institute for Public Policy Research; 2015. Available at: www.ippr.org/publications/powerful-people-reinforcing-the-power-of-citizens-and-communities-in-health-and-care

7. Monitor. Moving healthcare closer to home. IRRES 02/15. London: Monitor; 2015. Available at: www.gov.uk/government/uploads/system/uploads/attachment_data/file/459400/moving_healthcare_closer_to_home_summary.pdf

8. Bland J, Khan H, Loder J *et al*. *The NHS in 2030: a vision of a people-powered, knowledge-powered health system*. London: Nesta; 2015. Available at: www.nesta.org.uk/blog/nhs-2030-vision-better-future?gclid=CPSWmZ7VvMgCFSLnwgodNC4KzQ

9. Ofcom. *Internet Use and Attitudes: 2015 metrics bulletin*. London: Ofcom; 2015. Available at: http://stakeholders.ofcom.org.uk/market-data-research/other/research-publications/adults/media-lit-10years/

10. NHS. *Staffordshire and Stoke-on-Trent Five Year Strategic Plan 2014–19*. NHS; 2014. Available at: www.stokeccg.nhs.uk/

11. NHS Commissioning Assembly. *Technology Enabled Care Services: resource for commissioners*. London: NHSE; 2015. Available at: www.england.nhs.uk/wp-content/uploads/2015/04/TECS_FinalDraft_0901.pdf

12. National Information Board. *Workstream Roadmaps*. October 2015. Available at: www.gov.uk/government/publications/national-information-boards-workstream-roadmaps

13. NHS England. *Patient Online*. London: NHS England; n.d. Available at: www.england.nhs.uk/ourwork/pe/patient-online/

14. Bryan B, quoted in Armstrong S. Finally, the NHS goes digital. Or does it? *BMJ*. 2015; **351**: h3726. doi: 10.1136/bmj.h3726.

15. Greenhalgh T, Vijayaraghavan S, Wherton J *et al*. Virtual online consultations: advantages and limitations (VOCAL) study. *BMJ Open*. 2016; **6**: e009388. doi: 10.1136/bmjopen-2015-009388. Available at: http://bmjopen.bmj.com/content/6/1/e009388.full?eaf

16. European Code of Practice for Telehealth Services. *Telescope, 2015*. Available at: www.telehealth.global

17. Wherton J, Sugarhood P, Procter R *et al*. Co-production in practice: how people with assisted living needs can help design and evolve technologies and services. *Implement Sci*. 2015; **10**: 73. doi: 10.1186/s13012-015-0271-8.

18. Deloitte. *Mobile Consumer 2015: the UK cut; game of phones*. London: Deloitte; 2015. Available at: www.deloitte.co.uk/mobileuk/assets/pdf/Deloitte-Mobile-Consumer-2015.pdf

19. Stevenson D. Secure email pilot to cut 90% fax rate from care homes. *National Health Executive*. May/June 2015. p. 116.

20. Chambers R *et al. Tackling Telehealth: how CCGs can commission successful telehealth services*. London: *Inside Commissioning*; 2015. *Inside Commissioning and Simple Telehealth*. March 2014. Available at: http://offlinehbpl.hbpl.co.uk/NewsAttachments/GCC/Inside_Commissioning_Tackling_Telehealth.pdf

21. Deloitte. *Digital Health in the UK: an industry study for the Office of Life Sciences.* London: Deloitte; 2015. Available at: www.deloitte.co.uk/

22. Huxley C, Atherton H, Watkins J *et al*. Digital communication between clinician and patient and the impact on marginalised groups: a realist review in general practice. *Br J Gen Pract*. 2015; **65**: e813–21. doi: 10.3399/bjgp15X687853.

23. Ben-Zeev D, Drake R, Marsch L. Clinical technology specialists. *BMJ*. 2015; **350**: h945. doi: 10.1136/bmj.h945.

Chapter 2

Telehealth

Dr Ruth Chambers

What is telehealth?

Telehealth 'directly involves clinicians as an integral part of the service. ... It is used for regular monitoring of vital signs so that unusual activity can be detected before the situation becomes critical. Telehealth is an important tool for prevention and anticipatory care.'[1]

The terms 'e-health' and 'telehealth' are sometimes wrongly interchanged with the term 'telemedicine'. Like the terms 'medicine' and 'healthcare', the term 'telemedicine' is used to refer to the provision of clinical services while the term 'telehealth' can refer to clinical and non-clinical services such as medical education, administration and research. The term 'e-health' is often used, particularly in the UK and Europe, as an umbrella term that includes telehealth, electronic medical records and other components of health IT.

Describing the actual telehealth or telemedicine application, or distinguishing between them, will depend on their purpose and whether for instance the way of using the equipment renders it as a medical device. If the telehealth system is just a communication tool, it is not diagnostic, and it is not a medical device. Its success then depends on the user following the detail in the shared care management plan previously agreed with their health or social care professional.

The success of a telehealth application that is used to reinforce information in the management plan, therefore, is down to the way in which the communication changes the user's understanding, beliefs and behaviour in relation to the management of their health condition or improvement of their lifestyle habits.

Using telehealth for care of long-term conditions

Most clinicians would recognise that despite their best efforts, patients are for one reason or another unable to absorb all the information that the nurse or doctor would like to give them in a clinic visit. They may read it if it is handed to them on a leaflet, but often will not even do that, and instead rely on further advice from a health professional – or friend or unreliable media source. With a condition like chronic obstructive pulmonary disease (COPD), patients worry about their oxygen level (if they have a pulse oximeter to measure it), or the colour of their sputum or extent of breathlessness, and yet lack the confidence to manage on their own.

Telehealth readings can signal an impending crisis and enable the patient to seek help in advance of the deterioration of their condition; as well as their overseeing clinician(s) responding to relayed alerts. Patients may learn to recognise triggers that tend to derange the measures of their health that they are recording – such as stress triggering a raised blood pressure, or a rushed activity lowering their oxygen saturation level (SATS); then they can learn to avoid creating these triggers. Dual management plans agreed between the patient and their clinician(s) can allow the patient to initiate an intervention as previously agreed with their GP or practice nurse. For example, those with COPD can start taking standby prednisolone and/or antibiotic medication when there is a recognised deterioration in their condition.

Types of telehealth equipment

There are many suppliers of telehealth, so the type of equipment and nature of set-ups varies across the country and world, and from person to person. Telehealth can be set up so that monitoring systems allow patients with complex conditions to remain at home or be discharged early from hospital, and these require staff to triage readings sent in at a monitoring centre to trigger appropriate actions according to readings transmitted. In these types of systems, the patient is a passive recipient of care.

As clinicians have become more familiar with telehealth, there has been a move to cheaper and simpler equipment such as mobile phone texting that can give sufficiently good information to clinicians about patients' healthcare. The type and range of telehealth equipment should match patients' needs and preferences and be justified by: the risk of deterioration of their long-term condition(s), potential for a change in medication to prevent deterioration and availability of other interventions to reverse that deterioration and maintain them in better health.

Telehealth is delivered in many different ways across the world. Associated home-based sets of equipment typically include one or more of: weighing scales, sphygmomanometer, pulse oximeter, glucometer and ways of asking or relaying information about the patient's symptoms and condition and how they are feeling. More specialist additions are ECG, urine analyser or coagulation meter. In the UK popular telehealth methods are as follows:

1. SMS texting – there are many established systems. The Flo simple telehealth approach[2-5] has been taken up in many areas of the UK for clinical management, such as for hypertension, asthma, COPD, smoking cessation, cancer, pain etc., as well as reminders for medication and appointments. The clinician signing up the patient seeks their informed consent as well as their pledge to adhere to the agreed dual management plan and look after and return any associated equipment (e.g. pulse oximeter, sphygmomanometer). Exposing more people with lower risk levels of need to the benefits of simple telehealth solutions could help to encourage greater uptake of telehealth services for those with more complex needs. See www.simple.uk.net

2. Some telehealth systems are connected via telephone landline or mobile phone to a non-clinical triage (response) centre which requires specialist installation; others relay recordings via encrypted wireless and patients can take the equipment home or to work or away on holiday. Community matrons, mental health or district nurses may be contracted to respond appropriately to alerts from the triage centre if patients' readings are outside predetermined ranges; or they may monitor or act on the readings at regular intervals as part of a care package.

Portable and personal ECG monitors have been trialled for the early detection of cardiac ischaemia and arrhythmias generate alarm messages about the patient's heart function to a central web server that transmits messages in turn to the responsible clinician.

Widespread rollout of telehealth: Flo simple telehealth as an example

The evolution of the simple telehealth mobile phone texting service Florence (or Flo) has been developed in Stoke-on-Trent and the intellectual property is owned by the NHS. It has grown from applications relating to basic reminders for patients (e.g. to take medication) and self-reported information gathering (e.g. vital signs such as blood pressure), to enabling the provision of sophisticated clinical care underpinned by dual management plans agreed by clinician and patient. The evolution was driven by trials of clinical applications, such as that focused on improving clinical management of hypertension in general practice, funded by the Health Foundation.[2-5]

The initial evaluation of the clinical application for hypertension found that simple telehealth is an acceptable and effective tool in reducing patients' blood pressure in general practice settings[2.5]

Flo was developed to help patients to manage their long-term conditions or improve lifestyle habits in order to improve their state of health. Flo is different to other types of telehealth in many ways, because it is simple. Using text messaging, the only equipment required for many uses (e.g. reminders) is an ordinary mobile phone; although for some conditions monitoring equipment such as a sphygmomanometer may also be lent to patients. Flo sends reminder messages and advice messages to patients, and also asks the patient questions, and for some conditions asks the patient to text in their readings, such as those relating to their blood pressure. All text messages to and from Flo are free for the patient, as the NHS pays the cost. Patients love the support that they get from Flo and become more confident about co-managing their condition and less likely to contact their clinician unnecessarily.

EXAMPLE 2.1   Flo helps to get the balance right for palliative patients

Most palliative patients wish to remain independent for as long as possible. Sandra, a pioneering palliative care nurse champion, devised an independence pathway for the North Staffordshire area, whereby the patient is regularly contacted by Flo to ask if they are OK or would like help to ensure that they get timely assistance at home.

A good example is a patient who has had a tracheostomy and cannot communicate verbally but wishes to remain independent instead of receiving weekly district nurse visits. The patient reports feeling 'very supported by Flo' in lieu of district nurse visits and has the 'security and peace of mind' knowing that help is at hand when she needs it.

In another example, a community cancer lead suggested using Flo to increase the effectiveness of patient self-management throughout chemotherapy treatment. The Royal Stoke University Hospital already gives patients a thermometer to monitor their temperature after chemotherapy to detect early signs of possible infection. However, many patients struggle to follow the pathway advice and leave it too late to report signs of infection, resulting in higher costs from extra treatments and emergency admissions that could have been avoided. Patients also frequently forget to take anti-sickness and constipation drugs, resulting in avoidable demands on the community cancer team. Flo is offered to patients who are on a cancer treatment programme to assist with their temperature monitoring and medication compliance. Flo gives patients a sense of involvement and develops a self-care routine which heightens their awareness around possible infection and medication. This has resulted in earlier calls to the cancer centre, thereby triggering earlier interventions that prevent deterioration and decrease demand on the community team and avoid associated unplanned hospital admissions.

Flo requires commitment from the patient to make some effort to improve their own health, whether by making lifestyle changes or better adhering to treatment, or by regularly sending in texted responses to questions or readings of vital signs. Flo reinforces a dual management plan agreed between the clinician and the patient, but it is not a substitute for normal clinical care. The experience over the last three-year development period in primary, community, acute hospital and mental healthcare settings has been that patients gain more understanding of their condition through Flo, are more confident about their condition, do not feel the need to consult their clinicians as frequently, and their condition becomes more stable as they learn to adhere to advice or agreed interventions which previously were quickly forgotten.

EXAMPLE 2.2   Jeff's personal experiences of Flo simple telehealth for early dementia (given at a conference for doctors and nurses)

'My background – I:
- used to own and run a small business
- noticed that I was getting confused, forgetting technical procedures, appointments and lost my sense of direction
- have long history of high blood pressure, mini strokes, have a hole in the heart and angina
- went to my doctor and had further tests
- was diagnosed with MCI [mild cognitive impairment late last year].

'This left me in a confused state, unsure of the implications both personally and professionally.

'I was not sure of where to go for advice and help or what help and advice I needed.

'Luckily I was referred to the mental health and vascular well-being team and this is where I was introduced to Flo simple telehealth.'

'Flo and me
'I started on the Flo scheme and wore a camera to take snaps of my day – back in February 2015. I usually receive two Flo texts per day. Usually about 10.00 a.m. and 5.00 p.m. I have found these messages to be informative and very helpful.

'The subject content can vary, examples include remembering to stay hydrated, as water helps the brain to stay sharp and being thirsty distracts us. I remember to wear the Autographer camera. [Jeff was wearing a camera to take pictures of his day in automated ways at regular intervals so that he could combine the visual stimuli with support from Flo simple telehealth.]

'These messages may seem common sense but I can honestly tell you that they are of tremendous help and comfort to someone who can suffer from confusion and anxiety. Flo is not just a messaging service. It is a support system to those of us who find that day-to-day life is getting more challenging and subsequently feel unable to cope, which can lead to depression and other problems.

'I have in the past described it as resembling a friendly good-natured and trusted member of the family, who sends me a text just to help me through each day. Some days I am well enough to not take much notice of the message, but on my bad days they help to clear the fog and I can clearly see the way ahead. They make me think about the situation I find myself in and reaffirm the strategies and techniques that I have been taught by the excellent mental health team in order to make myself feel better and most importantly cope with my situation.

'Since I have been on the Flo programme I feel generally more confident, more able to cope and more confident about the future. I 100% believe in Flo and will do everything I can to support the system and promote its use. Please take it from me that I would not want to alter my daily routine (where I feel confident, in control and above all safe) to come here in front of people that I have not met before if it was not for the positive benefits that I have gained from Flo.'

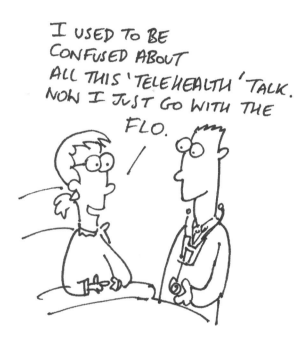

To make telehealth work at scale we need to emphasise and synchronise self-care and joint management (patient/clinician) across the local health economy with an agreed set of shared management plans to aid individual patients' self-management and clinician consistency with agreed local patient pathways.

Telehealth can be developed for a specific purpose such as the Modz for diabetes self-care. The children's version is designed as a motivational aid to keep blood glucose levels stable – as in Example 2.3.

EXAMPLE 2.3   mHealth for diabetes self-care

The readings from this touch screen blood glucose meter are sent automatically as text messages to a mobile phone (e.g. parent of child) and wirelessly to the Modz web cloud service where they can be accessed via the patient's healthcare team via Android and iOS devices. All test results, quantity of insulin or medication taken, meal contents, and exercise done can be logged and stored in the meter. The innovative design for children with diabetes is as an 'Angry Birds'-themed game-like monitoring system which motivates the child to achieve improved blood glucose levels through adhering to self-management guidance and plans. See: www.modz.fi or www.good4health.co.uk

So telehealth should be focused on the patient's needs and preferences. Box 2.1 captures some of the common needs in healthcare that telehealth might support – presented as an aide memoire.

BOX 2.1   Telehealth aide memoire for clinicians

Does this patient need:
✓ regular REMINDERS, e.g. for taking medication, to move to relieve pressure areas, to drink fluid, do exercises?
✓ regular MONITORING, e.g. blood glucose, temperature, blood pressure, pulse, pain score?
✓ MOTIVATIONAL MESSAGES to encourage compliance or adherence to their care plan, and increase their knowledge of their condition, e.g. diet, exercise, motivation?

If **YES** to any of the above, this patient may benefit from using telehealth.

Flo telehealth has been highlighted in this book because it is an effective exemplar of telehealth with much published evidence of its effectiveness to which the book authors have contributed. Box 2.2 contains many more examples of simple telehealth applications with Flo (or the landline version) for a wide range of long-term conditions or circumstances.

BOX 2.2 Range of Nottinghamshire-based Flo simple telehealth case studies

Nottinghamshire Assistive Technology Team led by Sian Clark
(Please note: all patients in these case studies have fictional names.)

Hypertension

Fraser is self-employed and was identified as being hypertensive during a health check. He was very anxious about the amount of time he would need to have off work in order to attend GP appointments. Fraser and his GP used Flo to monitor and titrate his medication. Flo was used to get baseline readings before anti-hypertensive medication was prescribed and then to collect blood pressure readings after Fraser began his medication.

Flo also prompted Fraser to book a telephone consultation with his GP to review his blood pressure readings. The GP reviewed the readings on his Flo clinical dashboard prior to the telephone consultation with Fraser and assessed his medication. Flo continued to request readings from Fraser until he was stable and then the frequency of requests was reduced.

The titration of Fraser's medication was much quicker due to the availability of blood pressure data to his GP. He has had no time off work, which reduced his anxiety, and he feels confident in managing his blood pressure depending on his readings, supported by the self-management plan that Fraser and his GP have agreed.

Pre-op hypertension

Hospital patients who are identified as hypertensive during their pre-op surgical assessment are sent home on Flo to remind them to send in their blood pressure readings twice a day for a week. This identifies patients who have white coat syndrome or genuinely have hypertension.

Cancelled operations due to hypertension are averted and patients who are identified as being hypertensive are referred to their GP with data which will help to initially titrate medication. Increasing numbers of GPs are continuing to use Flo to monitor and titrate their patients' medication. This speeds up the stabilisation of their condition and reduces the number of GP consultations required, which improves the patient experience and saves time and inconvenience.

The cost of lending blood pressure monitors and using Flo is £3.15 per patient. Seventy-five per cent of the patients put on Flo have been found to be hypertensive. More than 33 cancelled operations have so far been avoided.

Diabetes

Community nurses had been struggling to get Sid to comply with his diabetic care. Sid stopped recording his glucose levels and was taking his insulin in an ad hoc manner. He was also struggling with depression and looking after his alcoholic wife. They have a young family, and a neighbour had recently reported them to Social Services, stating that they felt the child was being neglected.

Since this event Sid became disengaged and lost motivation to manage his diabetes. When the nurse visited she was unable to titrate his insulin as there was no record about Sid's glucose levels. The nurse explained Flo to Sid and he was keen to try it and get his diabetes better controlled, particularly as he also expressed concerns that he was losing feeling in both his feet and had a recent fall.

Flo has been texting Sid three times a day every day for the past three weeks to remind him to test and submit his glucose readings and to take his insulin accordingly. The nurses now have access to his readings and can effectively titrate and support his insulin requirements remotely. Sid's readings are not yet stable and he has breached his parameters on a few occasions, but staff can now support him to manage and control his diabetes more effectively. The cost of using Flo with Sid is 72p per day.

Medication reminders

Patient story: 'I have ulcerative colitis which began when I was 11 years old and developed into cancer when I was 27 years old. In September 2010 my consultant prescribed an immunosuppressant which is supplied in a pen injection which I give myself every other Monday, i.e. fortnightly. Over the last couple of years my health has improved significantly and I am delighted with the results. It is important, however, to ensure that I give myself these injections at the same time every fortnight and I used to miss the scheduled time and even the correct day. Flo has totally removed this problem for me by sending me a text reminder at 6.30 p.m. every other Monday so I now take my medication at a regular time. Flo is such a simple process – just a text message reminder, but it has taken the onus off me to remember when to give myself my injection.'

(Cost = 8p a fortnight)

Using Flo landline (1)

A patient (aged 92 years old) had been discharged from hospital after a six week stay. The initial support for the patient ended and the patient needed to start ensuring she took her medication on her own. This was of great concern to the patient's family and Flo was discussed as an option. The patient now receives a telephone call from Flo to remind her to take her medication at set times agreed with the nurse, thus reassuring the family and giving the patient her independence back. Nearly two months post-discharge, the lady, who has early dementia, is taking her medication correctly and has had no admissions to hospital, whereas previously she had regular admission due to non-medication compliance.

Using Flo landline (2)

An anxious patient who has Parkinson's disease often forgot to take his night time medication before bed. His medication must be taken regularly to help control symptoms and he often combined the tablets with others the next day if forgotten. The patient was keen to try to use Flo and did start using a mobile phone, but he was often anxious about texting high blood pressure readings. The patient therefore swapped to a Flo landline and is now sending in his blood pressure readings as well as receiving the medication reminders. The patient is more in control of his care and feels better due to regularly taking his medication and receiving reassurance about his blood pressure readings.

COPD care plan

A COPD team is using Flo for patients to send in their oxygen saturation levels; if levels drop below the parameters set for the individual patient, Flo asks them for their cough, sputum and breathlessness scores. If required, Flo then asks the patient to contact the team. Patient contact has reduced as patients are managing their own condition better according to their pre-agreed care plan, and they feel reassured by Flo. Some patients who were previously quite anxious have reported reduced anxiety levels.

COPD: increasing use of rescue medication and averting hospital admissions

Patients using the Flo COPD protocol report that they feel much more in control of their health, are less anxious and know exactly when to take their rescue medication without having to contact their nurse or GP. Clinicians have highlighted that patients on this protocol would previously have been more likely to have been admitted to hospital with an exacerbation. Flo is highlighting early exacerbation and enabling early intervention, and therefore keeping these patients out of hospital.

COPD: a patient's view

A 55-year-old lady has been using Flo for six weeks. The community matron has indicated on the evaluation that the patient is managing their own health better and her contacts with the patient have been a lot fewer and more appropriate.

'Flo is a great help not only to me but to my husband who is my full-time carer. We both feel confident and reassured using Flo. We both think this service is an excellent idea. It allows not only me and my carers to keep a constant eye on my health but it also gives my community matron extra time to care more efficiently for people who may need her attention more. At the same time my community matron can also review the information I send daily to Flo any time which is very reassuring – an excellent scheme which should be continued.'

COPD: reducing exacerbations

An 81-year-old patient used Flo to manage his COPD with the help of his wife. His wife would take his readings and text them to Flo on his behalf. Since monitoring his COPD with Flo the patient feels happier, more confident and relaxed, and understands his condition better. With help from his wife, after eight weeks of using Flo, the patient learnt to text and now sends in his own readings. He feels confident to go out and is also more aware of when he would be better off staying at home and finds activities to keep himself busy. His wife has said that she worries a lot less about him when she is at work as she knows Flo will give him advice to follow. In the year before using Flo the patient had six exacerbations. The patient has now been using Flo for five months and has had no exacerbations.

Heart failure

The heart failure community nurses in Nottingham West and Nottingham North East are using Flo to monitor some of their patients' weight and blood pressure readings twice a week (age range 41–93 years). If the patient breaches set thresholds, Flo triggers messages advising the patient to contact their specialist nurse. Patient contact is becoming more appropriate and patients are reassured that they are be monitored in between nurse visits and if there are problems, Flo will pick these up and tell them what action to take. The team's home visits have halved since using Flo.

One of the heart failure nurses said: 'Flo is really working well – thanks. I have now had to increase one chap's weight readings to three times per week as his weight has gone up since last week, and he is clinically showing signs of deterioration; therefore I need to alter his medicines accordingly. Flo means that I don't have to go in three times per week. I still visit once per week, and as he gets worse I will have to go in more, but for now it is really helping me to gauge his condition.'

Heart failure: identification of atrial fibrillation (AF)

The Rushcliffe heart team has one specialist nurse covering 16 surgeries with a caseload of more than 80 patients. Flo is used to facilitate the clinics, enabling patients to be more proactive and helping to keep them out of hospital. Flo is offered to every patient at initial assessment. The nurse has reported how useful it is for monitoring the patients; it ensures that patients are being proactive in their management and provides reassurance for patients who report that they like taking control of their health.

An irregularity was picked up in one patient when using Flo to measure blood pressure using the monitors provided. This identified that the patient was in constant AF and resulted in the nurse liaising with the cardiologist with regard to cardioversion and appropriate treatment to be given.

Patients with co-morbidities

A community matron in Rushcliffe has been using Flo. For one patient in particular it has not only supported them but also their main carer. It has stopped their frequent calls to out-of-hours services. It has given his carers the confidence to use the agreed self-management plans, and it reassures the patient that although he is anxious and feels breathless his vital signs are actually stable. He is reassured that when he becomes unwell this will be picked up through Flo as his observations change.

Reducing numbers of community matron visits to a nursing home

A nursing home in Rushcliffe has begun a pilot using Flo to reduce the need for the community matron to visit unless vital signs readings indicate a visit is required. The carers, patients and family are all involved in the use of Flo. At a 'pre-go live' meeting with relatives and patients to explain how Flo works, some of the patients and relatives expressed the desire to send in readings. A review took place three months later and the programme was found to have been going well. Using Flo had identified three residents to the community matron who needed additional assessment, something which had not been picked up previously. One individual's blood pressure was very high, and the graph of Flo readings clarified this trend to the community matron and the staff at the home.

The staff felt reassured that they are giving the best quality care to the residents and requested that temperature monitoring be introduced if a resident appeared to be ill. Instead of needing a GP to visit, the staff can assess the individual using Flo and give the GP or community matron all the information about the resident and now know whether they have a raised temperature. Two more new residents have been added onto Flo. The team will continue to assess where Flo has reduced the need for a community matron or GP visit.

Each month patients are reviewed and a resident was recently identified as no longer requiring her medication for her long-term condition. The resident had always been reclusive and depressed. Flo readings identified she could stop her medication and since then she has been a changed lady – she is no longer depressed and is joining in and active in the home.

Further care homes are now utilising Flo to support the prevention of pressure sores and falls.

Supporting the gypsy, traveller and Romany (GTR) communities

The GTR communities are using Flo for medication reminders and weight management. The team has trained the gypsy traveller health ambassadors in Nottinghamshire, who are now signing up other GTRs. Given that 35% of GTR communities cannot read, they are using a special mobile phone app which will 'read' texts from Flo to users.

Weight management

Andy was morbidly obese and agreed to use Flo supportive messages and weight reading reminders to help him to lose weight. Unfortunately, when he attended the weight management clinic to sign up to Flo the scales provided were not of the appropriate specification to weigh him. Andy was extremely disappointed, but still keen to use Flo and suggested he could use the 'pay to weigh' scales in his local pharmacy once a week. The project change manager provided Andy with bariatric scales, after Andy admitted that weighing himself in public was very embarrassing and inconvenient. Having his own scales at home has provided further motivation for Andy to lose weight. Three weeks into using Flo, Andy has begun to lose weight on a weekly basis and is giving positive feedback on the motivational messages provided and suggesting additional ones that could be included to help others.

Weight management: supporting patients using Xenical
Practices are finding the Flo protocols for weight management are a useful and popular additional support tool for patients who are taking Xenical (orlistat) for weight reduction. One patient has already lost 3 stone (19 kg) in weight and feels continuously supported by Flo.

Interactive appointment reminders
The Child and Adolescent and Adult Psychiatry Clinics, based at Nottingham University Hospital, have used Flo as they had a did not attend (DNA) rate which at times was 55%. Flo reminds individuals about their appointments 1 week, 5 days, 3 days and then the day before their appointment, each time asking to confirm they are attending and if not giving a telephone number to ring to rearrange.

Of the patients now enrolled onto Flo, attendance is 100%. Patients are now asking for Flo to support them with reminders to pick up their prescriptions.

Interactive prompts for activities of daily living
The Social Care Asperger's team is using Flo with clients to check whether they have eaten a daily main meal. If they respond positively, they receive a positive message. If not, Flo texts them to encourage them to do so. If they answer negatively within a given time, Flo will text their key support worker or carer so that they can intervene as necessary. The individuals chosen reported forgetting to eat and are trying to remain independent and some have low body mass indices (BMIs). Using Flo is reducing the risks of carer breakdown within the families and also minimises the risk of admission to residential care. The individual with the lowest BMI has now put on 1 stone (6.3 kg) in weight since using Flo and has requested additional prompts. The team is also using Flo to prompt other reminders around an individual's activities of daily living with success. Service users have reported in the three-month review that Flo supports their needs. The support workers have also reported that Flo has meant that contact with these users has been more appropriate. Calculations for the nine individuals receiving prompts from Flo instead of home visits have estimated that the savings are around £300 per week.

Flo has also supported one client who was concerned about security; their story is told here: www.youtube.com/watch?v=ojRCGOna3Ug

Roundwood surgery
Roundwood surgery has taken a unique 'big bang' approach to using Flo for its

patients. Flo is used to support patients with COPD, heart failure, asthma, hypertension, weight management and diabetes. In the waiting area there is lots of information available for patients about Flo, including an enquiry box so that if they are interested in how Flo can help them to manage their condition or just relay a prompt for them to take their medication, they fill in a slip and pop it in the box. Practice team members review and then discuss with the patient whether Flo would be suitable for them to use.

The practice is now using Skype in conjunction with Flo to further exploit remote care monitoring and increase patient access to general practice.

One patient with COPD reported that he felt really supported by Flo in between practice visits, as he had never been sure when to take his rescue medication before, but now Flo will tell him when it is justified according to the messaged readings he texts in.

Visual impairment: supporting independence

A local practice is using Flo to support diabetic patients with hypertension. Once identified via the clinical system, these patients were invited to attend a Flo enrolment clinic. One patient, who was visually impaired, had support from a carer and could text using his own Braille mobile phone. He was keen to use Flo and was disappointed that he would need someone to help him with the blood pressure machine. The practice located a talking blood pressure machine and the patient is now taking his own readings and texting his readings to Flo.

Integrated health and social care

A Social Services team was using Flo to support a lady at home with medication reminders. This was successful and reassured the lady's daughter greatly that her mum was taking her blister pack medication. When the Social Services package finished, the daughter wanted her mum to continue to use Flo. The patient's GP agreed for the patient to be transferred to the practice to continue using Flo to enable the medication prompts to continue. So if any changes are required in the future to her medication, the practice will modify Flo messaging to continue this support.

Medication reminder: Parkinson's disease carer with Parkinson's too

Ron has Parkinson's disease and always gets his medication on time because his wife as his main carer supports him. However, his wife also has early stage Parkinson's disease and often forgets to take her own medication, which has resulted in her experiencing 'freezing' episodes. Flo has been set up to remind and prompt her to take her medication to ensure she can continue to care for Ron and herself.

Tell Flo and a technophobe

The team in Nottinghamshire were the first to deploy the new 'Tell Flo' app. A mobile phone is supplied for the patient with the 'Tell Flo' app installed and configured for their condition. It can be used for individuals who do not have the dexterity to text or as in this case do not have a mobile or landline phone. The Nottingham West heart failure team needed a way to better monitor the patient's heart failure, looking for early indicators of deterioration such as weight gain. The individual patient was quite apprehensive and did not like technology; however, they were willing to give it a go. The patient has now been successfully sending in their readings for the last two months and finds it very easy to use. 'Tell Flo' is so simple and improves the accessibility of Flo to all.

Post-stroke patient support

Pat is in her early fifties and has recently suffered a major stroke which has left her unable to speak and walk. Throughout her recovery her blood pressure has been high which may have been a contributing factor to her having a stroke. She was very anxious and concerned that her persistently high blood pressure would cause her to have another stroke.

During visits, the community matron suggested that the patient try Flo to send in weekly blood pressure readings. Pat was really pleased to start using Flo as she would be able to monitor her blood pressure and felt reassured and supported by the messages of advice she received from Flo. The community matron has now transferred this patient's Flo record to the patient's GP surgery so that the nurse and GP can monitor her readings closely. This has meant that Pat has been able to continue to use Flo with regular monitoring of her blood pressure; and her GP and nurse are able to titrate up her medication accordingly to try to stabilise her blood pressure and minimise the risk of another stroke.

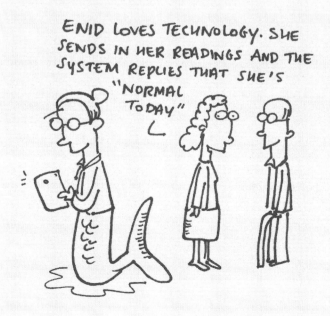

Parkinson's disease

A local Parkinson's disease group recently had a talk about Flo. Keith, who is the chairman, had difficulty speaking and was using a walking aid at the group talk. Keith volunteered as he was keen to see if Flo medication prompts would help him to ensure that he took his medication on time. After only three weeks of being registered on Flo, Keith called the oversight team and speaking clearly explained what a difference it had made to his health and that he was now sleeping at night too.

Diabetes landline insulin prompts

Terry often forgot to take his insulin at tea time. His wife would sometimes remember at bedtime and get up to go downstairs and administer Terry's insulin. Using Flo landline to issue a prompt at 6 p.m. each day has now ensured that they both remember that Terry must take his insulin at the right time, thus ensuring improved compliance and much better controlled glucose readings.

FAQs

Q1. Are there 'rules' as to how to use Flo simple telehealth? As a GP I don't think I'd have time to be looking at patients' texts as often as they are likely to send them in.

A. Because Flo is an adaptable tool, clinicians can decide how they want to use it. Community matrons tend to want to act on readings sent in by patients, and manage their workload according to the severity of individual patients' conditions, as indicated by readings from Flo. Most general practices use Flo as a shared care or self-care process where patients' management plans are reinforced by Flo. So in general practice, readings from Flo are monitored perhaps only once or twice a week or less, as Flo is helping the patients with self-management. Patients welcome the reassurance that they are fine and that their readings are within normal limits. They also like associated messages about their condition; for example, patients with COPD receive messages suggesting that if it's raining, they should do some exercise inside their house, such as walking up and down stairs, and patients with hypertension are advised to cut down on salt, or do regular exercise.

Q2. Does using a telehealth system make a patient with a long-term condition feel that they are being treated by a 'robot' rather than a healthcare practitioner who cares for them?

A. Someone with a long-term condition wants person-centred care – to be regarded as a person (not a condition) and to be treated holistically, so that all aspects of their health and social care are considered in one overall plan. So telehealth and other technology enabled types of care can support these person-centred approaches, supplementing but not replacing the clinician/carer-led care plan and reinforcing the shared management plan.

References

1. NHS Commissioning Assembly. *Technology Enabled Care Services: resource for commissioners.* London: NHS England; 2015. Available at: www.england.nhs.uk/wp-content/uploads/2015/04/TECS_FinalDraft_0901.pdf
2. Cottrell E, Chambers R, O'Connell P. Using simple telehealth in primary care to reduce blood pressure: a service evaluation. *BMJ Open.* 2012; **2**: e001391.
3. Cottrell E, McMillan K, Chambers R. A cross-sectional survey and service evaluation of simple telehealth in primary care: what do patients think? *BMJ Open.* 2012; **2**: e001392.
4. Chambers R, Cottrell E, Copeland P *et al.* Tackling Telehealth: how CCGs can commission successful telehealth services. *Inside Commissioning.* March 2014. Available at: http://offlinehbpl.hbpl.co.uk/NewsAttachments/GCC/Inside_Commissioning_Tackling_Telehealth.pdf
5. Cottrell E, Cox T, O'Connell P *et al.* Patient and professional user experiences of simple telehealth for hypertension, medication reminders and smoking cessation. *BMJ Open.* 2015; **5**: e007270.

Chapter 3

Why assistive technology should be a key part of health and social care services

Richard Haynes

Assistive technology (AT) can be used successfully by commissioners, care and support organisations, and the public in order to significantly improve outcomes in care of the elderly, frail, long-term or chronically sick, and disabled or impaired people. There is likely to be a type of AT that could be utilised to enable better care and support for all people, from those who have a low level of impairment, through to substantial and critical levels of need.

Organisations that support people are facing extraordinary challenges in meeting continuously rising needs in health and social care, in terms of absolute numbers, rising complexity and expectations. Economic pressures are driving changes so that resources are used to achieve improved outcomes in health and well-being within budgetary constraints.

Social pressures create a further burden on an already financially challenged system. People have increasing expectations of the quality and extent of care they think they should receive. As technology evolves and becomes more main-streamed, some people will expect such technology to be made available from statutory organisations such as local authorities. These pressures are prompting organisations to consider ways that people can increasingly help themselves and be more self-reliant and independent. Embedded within the Care Act[1,2] is a new emphasis on prevention and well-being: acting to prevent crises that might otherwise trigger admissions to hospitals or care homes. Technology enabled care services (TECS) play an important role in addressing these challenges.

Legislation and policy

The Care Act[1] puts well-being and prevention at the heart of all care services. The Act also places accountability on statutory authorities to try to support people for as long as possible at home or in their preferred place of care. Important UK legislation, regulation, and White Papers that impact on AT include the Care Act 2014; the Human Rights Act 1998;[3] the Equality Act 2010;[4] and initiatives such as Think Local Act Personal,[5] *Valuing People*, and *Independence, Well-being and Choice*.[6, 7]

Specifically, the key impact on AT strategy of the Care Act,[1,2] which brings together a key number of other elements of regulation, includes the following:

1. Enablement of more options for choice of where care is provided, closer to family. Services should consider interventions for prevention at every stage and interaction (which includes domiciliary as well as residential and nursing care guidance).
2. Prevention is a continuous activity and AT should be considered at all times, i.e. if equipment is not suitable, domiciliary care providers could raise this and not wait for reviews which are rarely up to date on equipment. Contracts should reflect this. There is also a possible role for home care providers to review equipment, which would also reduce some pressures on care management and assessment teams.
3. Free provision of minor aids and adaptations (covers most AT fall aids) up to the value of £1000. (If this is to be done effectively though services for community equipment, telecare, telehealth and AT should not be siloed.)

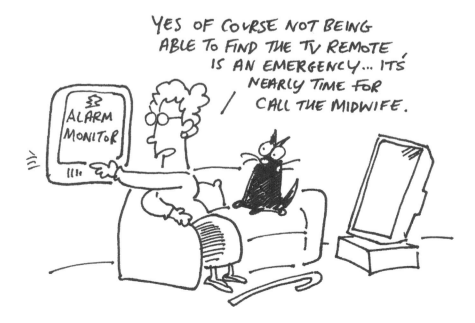

4. Provision of AT to support or enable people to attend college, school or hold a job, e.g. by using GPS for safer travel or smartphone with prompts or timetabling.

5. Appropriate training or qualifications, and trusted assessor schemes, that are in place in councils and NHS providers. Councils and NHS providers could delegate or commission other providers, such as patient groups and user-led organisations, to assess others for equipment needs (new or existing).

6. Moving AT equipment along with the person regardless of cost. Providers and services need to be aware of this. Telecare or AT is the person's own equipment and is effectively on long-term loan.

7. Consideration of implications for training the workforce in relation to AT including any interaction with providers' ICT systems. The key challenge seems to be the upskilling of the workforce and generating of new behaviours, so that staff are more creative, with lateral thinking.

Defining assistive technology (AT)

Technologies are often described collectively as 'assistive technology' in the context of impairment and disability. It could be argued that the term 'assistive technology', or 'electronic assisted living technology' (eALT), reinforces traditional or outmoded clinical models. The importance of citizenship and people taking a more active part in society means that patients should be recognised as experts in their own right. AT should be defined and framed within a context of the social model of disability (SMOD), where the SMOD is at the heart of personalisation that is widely accepted by service users and patients. Personalisation and the SMOD are also enshrined implicitly within key pieces of UK legislation, regulation, and White Papers.[1-6]

> A great example of SMOD and technology applied in a highly personalised way is a preferred music protocol employing iPods and iTunes called Music & Memory and is featured in the the international award winning film *Alive Inside*; watch the trailer here: www.aliveinside.us/ and visit http://musicandmemory.org/ for more information on the use of technology in dementia care, mental health and learning disabilities.

The following description offers a good framework for what is meant by AT:

> any item, piece of equipment, product or system, whether acquired commercially, off the shelf, modified or customised, that is used to increase, maintain or improve the functional capabilities of individuals with cognitive, physical or communication disabilities.[8]

Where earlier definitions are mostly functional, a user-led definition, facilitated by FAST at The King's Fund,[9] additionally frames independence and associated SMOD as: '... any product or service designed to enable independence for disabled and older people'.

This could be, for example, to increase opportunities for employment, training or education (as implied in the Care Act,[1,2] or simply having fun, increasing access to local leisure services and thereby being more active, and improving mental, physical and social well-being.

Maximising the benefits for as many stakeholders as possible

The benefits of full implementation of AT are:

1. Improved health and well-being
2. Effectiveness (quality, process improvement, employment relations)
3. Legal (including policy and regulatory guidance)
4. Pleasure (increasing fun, employment, education and training for staff and customers and carers)
5. Safeguarding (improving security, health and safety)
6. Management (increasing flexibility, improving decision making, management processes and strategic fit, i.e. as part of a programme or corporate transformation)
7. Economic (efficiency, savings and income generation).

These categories are represented by the acronym H-E-L-P-S M-E, as shown in Table 3.1 (*see* p. 44).

Innovation

New possibilities are continually emerging through new innovations including smart home technology, mobile and web apps and devices, brain–machine interfaces, robotics and 3D printing. Creativity and lateral thinking addressing needs are required at every level of an organisation and each step of the care pathway.[10] So new technologies should not be overlooked nor services be left behind by under exploiting technology.

Beyond telecare and telehealth

An extended definition of AT could include and encompass the following features:

1. AT uses any art, skill and craft to make, modify and use tools. Some companies provide highly bespoke-tailored technologies, funded by voluntary contributions, which are excellent examples of what can be accomplished

TABLE 3.1 H-E-L-P-S M-E

Health and well-being	• Better proactive management of mental health – early intervention before escalation • Better medicines optimisation • Improved outcomes in reduction of falls • Increased social inclusion and reduced isolation • Support for people with mental or learning impairment, cognitive function, e.g. memory problems, budgeting • Enabling people to access other opportunities in areas they value and to be more independent
Effectiveness (quality of service, process improvement, HR)	• Improved perception of services through what is seen as additional elements (rather than reductions) by service users, families, carers and care management • Career development path for professionals ranging from National Vocational Qualification (NVQ) to postgraduate levels of study, on-the-job stimulation and challenge, and opportunities to improve outcomes for people • Better support for carers so that they can continue to provide care for longer
Legal (policy, regulatory)	• Better compliance with well-being, prevention and assessment components of the Care Act[1] • Meet specific requirements as outlined in supporting regulatory information
Pleasure (increasing fun, employment, education, training)	• Use of technology can be fun • AT can increase opportunities to work, take up education and training, through increased independence or by supporting outcomes in both functional and instrumental activities of daily living
Safeguarding (security, health, safety)	• Improving people's security, e.g. through safer walking with GPS devices, better compliance with medication, or safer moving and transfers • Better visibility in people's patterns of daily living to ensure that vulnerable people are sleeping and eating; providing solutions where routines fall outside of safe and normal patterns
Management (flexibility, decision making, management processes, strategic fit)	• More flexible responses to rising need where provision of technology reduces a person's dependence on resources or others' face-to-face support for which it can be hard to recruit and retain staff • AT lifestyle monitoring systems aid safer, more accurate, and usually more cost-effective outcomes to assessments
Economic (efficiency, income)	• Increased efficiencies through use of AT, so preventing, delaying and reducing unnecessary home care spend, enhancing supported living and residential care placements • Increased competitiveness as a provider, where a provider markets its offer on the basis of greater use of AT • Income through commercial offers generated

through recognising service users and patients as equal partners. REMAP, for example, has designed and provided devices including: those to help people with quadriplegia read books, generic wheelchair mounting systems for physically disabled parents to take children with them on their wheelchairs and Xbox controllers for disabled people.[11] Another great example is Fixperts, which provides an approach to working in a unique way with service users, demonstrating how increased engagement of users and equal and meaningful involvement in the design process overcome a range of challenges.[12]

2. AT creatively applies knowledge to solve challenges of providing care, by involving people and machines to accomplish goals. There is scope through current referrals to and assessments of health or social care to be more creative and innovative by working with other disciplines; for example, in housing for preemptively adaptable houses (as opposed to being simply reactively adapted); blue light services; and mechanical, electrical and software engineers.[13]

3. AT is any item, product or system that can be acquired commercially, off the shelf or modified or customised. We are massively underutilising the capacity that exists within the local economy and people's aspirations to use less stigmatised, more mainstream technology (which has as much to do with the experience and patient or service user journey as it does the type or purpose of technology).

4. AT increases, maintains or improves functional cognitive, physical or communication abilities and consequently increases (in some instances) a person's independence.

5. AT enables greater opportunities for improved physical, mental and social well-being through enhanced prospects of work, education and training as well as more leisure time and pleasure. This is sometimes with reduced environmental costs, which can in some cases achieve more efficient use of energy and reduced carbon emissions.

How can e-assistive living technology (eALT) help people?

eALT can provide greater choice and control for people over their own lives. For example, it can support people in making decisions on where they wish to live (which is a new statutory obligation placed on local authorities in the Care Act[1]).

eALT can also enable people to live in their own home for longer with increased confidence and safety, and in many cases reduce the need for unplanned care, which can come at great social and economical costs to the person requiring care and their families. Many early and traditional services have focused on the needs of older people (and to a lesser degree people with dementia[8]). eALT is now widely recognised as being of benefit to adults and carers of any age as well as children, and can play a key role for people in their everyday lives. For examples of how eALT can help people with learning disabilities (LD), the Hft, a charity supporting people with LD, has a helpful 'virtual' smart house (available online at www.hftsmarthouse.org.uk/). There is also a useful website for people looking for eALT solutions who care for someone with, or who themselves have, dementia: www.atdementia.org.uk/

eALT can support people in a number of ways by:

1. ensuring that minor events do not turn into crises
2. making sure that when something significant happens, an alert can be raised and an appropriate response is provided promptly
3. supporting better quality and more efficient assessments and early interventions, through improved supportive planning; for example, by monitoring patterns of daily living
4. analysing responses to detect symptoms which may have a more serious underlying cause, and initiating earlier interventions to prevent a greater need occurring
5. providing quick and efficient means for people to be connected and included in society, thus reducing isolation and loneliness.

Lack of uptake

Reasons for the lack of uptake of AT include the following:[14]

1. Lack of awareness of what telecare and telehealth equipment is available and how it might be used.
2. Difficulties in discussing AT with potential service users and their families.
3. Lack of integration into processes as part of initial assessments and ongoing reassessments or reviews.

Technology needs to be personalised and tailored to the individual

Technology is not a 'one size fits all' solution. The person's needs should always be fully considered in order that eALT solutions are personalised and tailored to the individual. Falls detection is a good example. Thirty per cent of people who have a fall lie undetected for at least one hour[15] and of these people, half will die within six months.[16] A fall detector does not prevent a fall but can clearly help carers to respond more quickly to reduce the likelihood of incurring greater emotional, social and economic costs. Fall detectors have been shown to give users greater confidence so that they are more active and independent around their house or garden.[17,18]

How fall detectors are set up, used and calibrated determine their success. Involvement of the person is crucial in the setting up and use of detectors in order that they are used properly, and do not generate too many false readings (it is impossible not to have some false readings), balanced against the need to provide useful alerts. The application and type of use, for example, the level of activity of the individual, is critical in the correct choice and calibration of a fall detector; so is how the device is worn, which may come down to personal preference – a key factor in the likelihood of adoption? The implications for care and support organisations are how do they best assess people, involve service users in the process as equals, and what range of equipment do they procure or commission?

Other significant barriers to the uptake of AT (as well in many cases a lack of service user involvement) need to be understood, or else existing and new service models risk being highly inefficient. If a service has less than 50% of its users continuing to use equipment provided (where 80% use is not unusual[14]), and is not reviewing or finding out why, there is clearly a great deal of effort going into generating activity that leads to low levels of uptake, and this is simply inefficient.

In developing an AT service, you need to understand the reasons for high numbers of people commonly abandoning eALT and seek solutions that overcome the main barriers.

Telecare uptake remains very low. Traditional telecare (the most basic level of a pendant or pull cord system with a community alarm) is taken up by less than 3% of the population of people over the age of 65 years, who could otherwise benefit from AT. Nationally, community equipment in general is supporting just 40% of the population who could benefit.[19] Not using some of this equipment means that, for some, carers' lives are more difficult, and service users are missing out on opportunities for an enhanced quality of life, and both service users and caregivers are at risk of an injury or further decline in their independence or well-being that might have otherwise been avoided. There is an excellent video called *Uninvited Guests*, available online, which provides insights into some of the possible frictions between users and technology and potential barriers: www. superflux.in/work/uninvited-guests. After watching the video, it's worth asking yourself: What did the person really need? How could this have been picked up better on an assessment? How could the person have been involved more? What technologies, including those from the mainstream, might have been more useful?

The MATCH project (Mobilising Advanced Technologies for Care at Home) focused on barriers to the uptake of home care technologies.[20] This included a variety of stakeholders in telecare, including older users, their friends and family, health and social care professionals, and policy makers. The main barriers to the uptake of telecare in the UK were found to be: lack of availability of resources, limited awareness raising and education, too little focus on personalisation; acceptance issues; limited evolution of services; and ethical and legal issues.

Return on investment and value for money for citizens

If the challenges and barriers can be addressed, AT represents very good value for money for citizens and those funding provision of care, by providing a return on investment.

One national case study of a sample of 240 users, based on real costs at the time of commissioning, found that for every £1 spent on telecare, £3.82 was saved on traditional care, and for people for whom telecare was a direct replacement for traditional care, £12.60 was saved. Seven people (3%) out of the 240 sample of users were diverted from residential care.[21]

In a separate independent evaluation of a Scottish telecare programme, savings were reported as: 546 000 care home bed days, 109 000 hospital bed days through facilitated discharges and avoided unplanned admissions, 48 000 nights of sleepover/wakened night care and 444 000 home check visits. Overall, the gross value of the programme funded with around £7 million capital and revenue support delivered efficiencies of approximately £78.6 million at current prices over the 5-year period.[22]

Service user take-up

Abandonment and refusal rates of telecare and AT can be as high as 80%.[23] Rather than the problem being an issue with the nature and stigma of AT products, one of the causes thought to be contributing to the low uptake is with a 'one-size fits all' approach to telecare schemes. Such an approach typically involves handing responsibility for the service over to a single supplier, and thus seeing it as a simple infallible solution rather than a more complex scenario of culture and change management with collaborative working by health and social care professionals. This is further compounded by a lack of investment in the workforce, where commissioning a single entity to take on telecare is doomed. The key to greater adoption could therefore be in investment in the workforce and greater involvement from service users and patients where, through their engagement, many of the barriers found in the MATCH study[20] could be addressed by improved patient knowledge and awareness, and by networking between patients or service users and carer groups.[24]

Greater user involvement leads to better take-up, more useful application of technology, increased satisfaction and more efficient services

In one study of 136 users of hearing aids (and 149 users of manual wheelchairs), researchers found an association between greater involvement of users in AT (for example, in understanding personal needs, wishes or ongoing use) and far higher levels of adoption and usefulness of AT.[25] The challenge remains, though, to reach and engage people who might be potential users of AT, before their needs escalate.

People are not 'hard to reach', rather services are hard to access

The notion of groups of people being assumed to be 'hard to reach', for example people with reduced mental capacity through LD; people with mental health problems, dementia and of different ethnicity and cultural background, is a contested and ambiguous term.[26] Is the limited use of AT services by 'hard to reach' groups because the service seems hard to access for those groups of people? For example, there is (rightly) a focus in most public sector organisations on provision of digital care, so that people use efficient digital means of engagement as an alternative or adjunct to usual care. Many services are focusing efforts on digital offers and information, at the cost sometimes of face-to-face communication. But the target audience of people who are least well, physically, mentally and socially, or have at least one disability or impairment, are also likely to be more vulnerable, less financially secure and consequently (due to social factors and finances) least likely to have a computer or Internet access at home. And these are two essential technologies that many organisations are relying on to deliver information to people to prevent, delay or reduce a need.

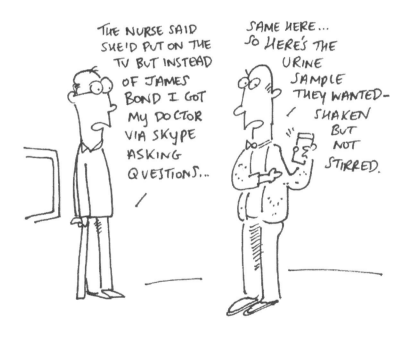

So how can we apply learning from the evidence to improve provision of AT?

Organisations should:

1. invest more in activities that promote awareness, and work with communities to build capacity and resources
2. develop AT as a 'brand' which is desirable and not stigmatised. AT needs to be perceived more as a 'Gucci' or 'James Bond' style, so people want it, like the next Apple product
3. tailor solutions to people to be person led rather than technology led
4. involve service users and carers as far as possible in service design and provision, including assessments; Fixperts is a good example of this approach[12]
5. make the pathways simpler and less confusing, and promote the different channels of provision (supporting self-help) more widely. Resolve issues where pathways are confusing, such as where conflicting levels of funding exist from different local providers, depending on the type of device and health or social care setting
6. develop the wider workforce, in particular in the ethical aspects of AT and provide a framework for better assessments; see *Ethical Frameworks for Telecare Technologies for Older People at Home (EFORTT)* for examples of ethics applied in the development of eALT[27]
7. better understand and learn from the reasons for people's refusals and abandonment of AT, so that other alternatives can be considered where one intervention has not worked.

Taking AT forward as an organisation or local health and social care economy

Your broad aims should be to:

- move towards more person-centred outcomes and more cost-efficient and -effective services; developing patient reported outcomes measures (PROMs) for AT may be a good thing to consider
- align AT range and availability with population needs on a demographic basis as well as on an individual basis
- mainstream AT into first contact, information, advice, guidance and care management and assessment processes, broader systems of service delivery, performance management and public involvement and engagement
- develop procurement and market-shaping activities so that there is an AT offer for people who are not necessarily covered by statutory care on a preventative basis, as well as through normal supply chain routes for statutory areas[28]
- identify the strategic needs of ICT systems to support implementation and ongoing use and monitoring of AT uptake, including performance

management (*see* ADASS, *Developing a Series of Metrics for Telecare*, online at: www.adass.org.uk/uploadedFiles/adass_content/policy_lead/standards_ and_performance/Metrics%20for%20telecare%2030%209%2014%20final. pdf).

The desired outcomes may not be achievable, however, if your service redesign is purely cost driven or targeted at a more corporate level. The challenges that the demographics of local populations present are well understood. It is less well appreciated that AT can support a more diverse group of individuals, other than older people or people with a physical disability. For example, AT can support people with mental impairments arising from LD, dementia, mental health and also drug and alcohol dependency, child carers and victims of domestic abuse.

There is some evidence that AT and telecare initiatives have not delivered expected savings, in contrast to a lot of other good qualitative and quantitative evidence of perceived benefits and increased independence. If AT is broadly applied with creativity and with care, it can enable people to not only be safer and more independent but also to be part of society and contribute to it. This is a good example of the application of the SMOD approach described earlier.

If an organisation's primary aim is to save money, it may be that a more inclusive view of a wider range of stakeholders and their needs may lead to the design and delivery of more efficient services. AT can benefit a diverse group of people, improving outcomes for carers as well as service users or patients. Providers who demonstrate good practice in AT may market and promote their services or organisations on this basis. AT can also help care professionals in achieving improved decision making. Commissioners and people who pay charges may want to make the most efficient use of the limited number of support hours available from an increasingly limited labour market for paid carers.

Building a good solid business case, and secure support, requires the buy-in of multiple stakeholders, as opposed to the business case being built purely on efficiencies alone, if the project is to be successfully implemented and embedded, and not just approved.

FAQs

Q1. What are the major driving forces behind the impetus for the implementation of any substantive TECS such as AT and telecare?

A. They are:

- personalisation
- changing attitudes
- demographics
- government spending.

Q2. Are there any good courses you can recommend to learn more about AT?

A. Organisations thinking about the development of their workforce may wish to consider investment in staff at either a foundation or postgraduate level in AT; see, e.g. www.coventry.ac.uk/course-structure/2014/faculty-of-health-and-life-sciences/postgraduate/assistive-technology-msc/

Q3. My customers and staff say using AT is 'a bit big brother'. Do they have a point?

A. Yes and no. It depends on how the client is involved, and whether they have capacity. How have ethics been considered? The Beauchamp and Childress model on clinical ethics may be useful as well as the initiative at Lancashire University on ethics of AT (EFORTT).[27] An AT intervention may be restrictive but could just be the least restrictive and most beneficial intervention to include in the care plan for the person or their caregiver. The semantics and language used, which indicates the use and emphasis on who it benefits, may be subtle and important too. For example, think about how GPS is presented as ether: 'a GPS tracker to track you' compared to 'a GPS locator to primarily help you to locate yourself if lost, and summon help if needed'. How have people been involved, how is information collated (through lifestyle monitoring systems for example) and presented and for whose benefit?

Q4. How much do I have to know about the technology to use AT?

A. It's more important to be curious and think creatively and laterally than it is to know all there is to know technically about AT. With a curious mind, and access to Google, Bing, Amazon, eBay and the high street, there is very little that has not been invented or possible, and even where something might not have been invented, organisations like REMAP can help.

Q5. How will AT for my patients or service users be paid for?

A. A lot of the best AT equipment is standalone and inexpensive. Much of it is easily available to anyone from normal retail channels. For people requiring more complex interventions or more expensive solutions, the Care Act has provision for up to £1000 of minor aids (for which AT is one such example) and adaptations for a client, free of charge and provided preventatively from Social Services. Beyond this cost, if the AT is a required intervention to meet an unmet need, there may be good reasons to consider this as non-traditional service-orientated provision (again a requirement in the Care Act, considering interventions such as the provision of Internet access or ICT).

References

1. Department of Health (DH). *Care Act 2014: statutory guidance for implementation*. London: DH; 2014. Available at: www.gov.uk/government/publications/care-act-2014-statutory-guidance-for-implementation

2. Social Care Institute for Excellence. *How is Wellbeing Understood under the Care Act?* Available at: www.scie.org.uk/care-act-2014/assessment-and-eligibility/eligibility/how-is-wellbeing-understood.asp

3. Human Rights Act 1998. Available at: www.legislation.gov.uk/ukpga/1998/42/contents

4. Equality Act 2010. Available at: www.legislation.gov.uk/ukpga/2010/15/contents

5. www.thinklocalactpersonal.org.uk/

6. Department of Health (DH). *Valuing People: a new strategy for learning disability for the 21st century*. White paper. Cm 5086. London: DH; 2001. Available at: www.gov.uk/government/uploads/system/uploads/attachment_data/file/250877/5086.pdf

7. Department of Health (DH). *Independence, Well-Being and Choice: our vision for the future of social care for adults in England*. London: DH; 2005. Available at: www.gov.uk/government/uploads/system/uploads/attachment_data/file/272101/6499.pdf

8. Marshall M. *ASTRID: a guide to using technology within dementia care*. London: Hawker Publications; 2000.

9. FAST. *FAST: Definition of the term 'Assistive Technology'*. London: FAST; n.d. Available at: www.fastuk.org/about/definitionofat.php

10. Faife D. Reflections on developing an assistive technology/telecare service as a model for change management, creative thinking and workforce development. *Hous Care Support*. 2008; **11**(4): 34–42.

11. remapleics.org.uk

12. Fixperts.org. *Fixperts*. 2015. Available at: http://fixperts.org/fixfilms/

13. Woonlabo.be. *UD Woonlabo*. 2015. Available at: www.woonlabo.be/en/node/449

14. Sanders C, Rogers A, Bowen R *et al*. Exploring barriers to participation and adoption of telehealth and telecare within the Whole System Demonstrator trial: a qualitative study. *BMC Health Serv Res*. 2012; **12**(1): 220.

15. Fleming J, Brayne C. Inability to get up after falling, subsequent time on floor, and summoning help: prospective cohort study in people over 90. *BMJ*. 2008; **337**: a2227.

16. Wild D, Nayak USL, Issacs B. How dangerous are falls in old people at home? *Br Med J* (Clin Res Ed). 1981; **282**(6260): 266–8.

17. Holliday N. *Fall detectors – what do users want?* Coventry: Health Design Technology Institute. 2012. Available at: http://goo.gl/LNbzOr

18. Various research undertaken by Coventry University on falls. Available at: www.coventry.ac.uk/

19. Capital Ambition Project Proposal. *Transforming Community Equipment Services in London*. 2015. p. 7. Available at: http://intranet.londoncouncils.gov.uk/London%20Councils/Item6aCapitalAmbitionreportJIPProgrammeOutcome17.1.doc

20. Clark J, McGee-Lennon M. A stakeholder-centred exploration of the current barriers to the uptake of home care technology in the UK. *J Assist Technol*. 2011; **5**(1): 12–25.

21. Department of Health Archives. 2010. *Putting People First – Transforming Adult Social Care: efficiencies in telecare*. Available at: http://webarchive.nationalarchives.gov.uk/+/www.csed.dh.gov.uk/_library/Resources/CSED/CSEDProduct/CSED_Case_Study_Essex_final.pdf

22. Newhaven Research. *The Telecare Development Programme in Scotland 2006–11.* 2015. Available at: www.jitscotland.org.uk/wp-content/uploads/2014/07/TDP-Final-Evaluation-July-2011.pdf

23. Subramanian U, Hopp F, Lowery J *et al.* Research in home-care telemedicine: challenges in patient recruitment. *Telemed J E Health.* 2004; **10**(2): 155–61.

24. Beresford P. *Beyond the Usual Suspects: towards inclusive user involvement.* London: Shaping Our Lives; 2013.

25. Borg J, Larsson S, Östergren P *et al.* User involvement in service delivery predicts outcomes of assistive technology use: a cross-sectional study in Bangladesh. *BMC Health Serv Res.* 2012; **12**(1): 330.

26. Flanagan S, Hancock B. 'Reaching the hard to reach': lessons learned from the VCS (voluntary and community sectors); a qualitative study. *BMC Health Serv Res.* 2010; **10**(1): 92.

27. Department of Sociology. *Ethical Frameworks for Telecare Technologies for older people at home (EFORTT).* Lancaster: Lancaster University; 2015. Available at: www.lancaster.ac.uk/efortt/

28. NHS England. *Launch of Technology Enabled Care Services (TECS) Resource for Commissioners.* Available at: www.england.nhs.uk/ourwork/qual-clin-lead/tecs/

Other resources to view

1. *Uninvited Guests*: www.superflux.in/work/uninvited-guests
2. GPS shoes: www.youtube.com/watch?v=Feutw61nhPA
3. *Alive Inside*: www.aliveinside.us/
4. Hft Virtual Smart House: www.hftsmarthouse.org.uk/
5. AT Dementia site: www.atdementia.org.uk/
6. Web-based assessment for falls: https://cele.coventry.ac.uk/fallcheck/?page=about

Chapter 4

Applying telecare and assistive technology in practice

Jim Ellam

Telecare is support and assistance provided at a distance using technology. It involves the continuous, automatic and remote monitoring of users through the use of sensors which allows people to continue living in their own home, at the same time minimising risks such as preventing a fall. This chapter focuses on how community alarms and telecare work, and where and how they can be used. It also looks at commonly used standalone technologies with examples of how telecare can support independence and assessment processes. These solutions can underpin assessment processes and offer ongoing support and reassurance for informal carers, friends and family.

Assistive technology (AT) is 'any device or system that allows an individual to perform a task that they would otherwise be unable to do, or increases the ease and safety with which the task can be performed'.[1]

The FAQs at the end of this chapter provide links to sources of further information, useful video clips and some simple to use online guides to help find suitable AT options for the service user and their needs that you are considering. This short video demonstrates some of the technologies available and outcomes that they can support: www.youtube.com/watch?v=mq_AKfjFkDo

Assistive technology as an enabler

There is no one magic product that will suit all people and all situations. The use of AT is appropriate for everyone and it should not be considered as simply a direct replacement for personal contact and carers' support. It should be seen as enabling people to lead their own lives and not restrict their movement and independence. Ethical issues relating to AT and independence have been considered by the Social Care Institute for Excellence; see www.scie.org.uk/publications/ataglance/ataglance24.asp

Personalisation is well established within social care and is now being embraced by the NHS. The shift from a service-based approach to one that focuses on the individual and their outcomes requires new ways of working, so valuing the insights and engagement of the individual recipient of health and care services.

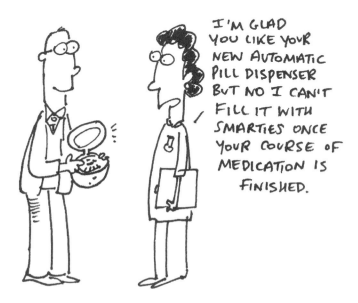

Traditionally services have been based or built around visits to or from care professionals. Technology offers a range of options to work differently, freeing up carers' time for what is required and offering a more flexible, personalised and cost-effective service to deliver improved clinical and social outcomes.

Technology is increasingly integrated into our everyday lives. We use technology for entertainment, food preparation, communication and transport. The technology we use supports our ability to shape the outcomes that we want. However, on the whole, care professionals do not routinely consider the use of technology for delivery of health and care services to support people's ability to self-care and enable greater independence, choice and control in their lives.

In the UK the use of technology is common:[1]

- more than seven in ten people use technology to either bank, pay bills, shop or communicate
- six in ten people use technology in leisure activities (61%) or travel (58%)
- 62% use social networking such as Facebook or Twitter
- only 2% of the population say that technology doesn't feature in their lives.

But when the public was asked about the different ways in which they used technology in their lives, health and care came in last place.[2] Fewer than one in three people (30%) use technology to support health and care – coming behind banking, shopping, communicating, social networking, leisure, travel, work, learning and education.

In an 'Age of Austerity' with significant constraints on health and care budgets, service redesign must address the pressures that our demographic population changes are creating with the increasing demand for services.[3] NHS England is promoting technology enabled care services (TECS) at a national level to transform healthcare delivery, yet TECS still appear to be a secondary consideration compared with traditional care services, rather than being considered as a key enabler of effective delivery of care.

For health and care professionals AT can support the assessment process, helping to monitor daily living activities which when interpreted enhance their understanding of a person's abilities and areas of dependency. It can help people to self-manage their care and conditions and can identify when and where carers' input is required rather than carers visiting people 'just in case'. This helps free up carers' time so that resources can be redirected for those people who most need it.

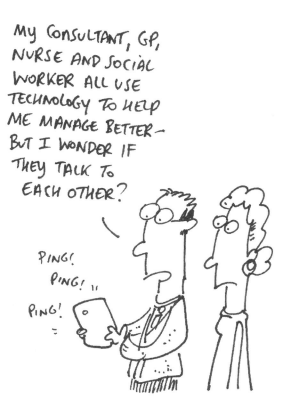

Telecare technology

Using community alarms and telecare technology can help people of any age and ability to live independently, safely and securely in their own home. It can also give family and friends peace of mind that they can be contacted in an emergency. Additionally, carers' pagers can be provided which alert live-in family carers only when help is needed, allowing them some respite from their caring role. This can be particularly helpful during the night when onsite carers can sleep soundly with the assurance that the telecare pager will alert them when support is required; for example, if someone gets out of bed, approaches the door exit, has an epileptic seizure or fall etc. While commonly used by around 1.8 million people within domestic settings and housing schemes in the UK, there is still limited take-up in care homes and hospital settings that provide care for the most vulnerable people.

The Disabled Living Foundation provides a useful and regularly updated fact sheet which offers practical help and advice to consider in relation to community alarms and telecare: www.dlf.org.uk/factsheets/factsheet_telecare.pdf

A community alarm or care call system links the person at home to a 24-hour monitoring centre through a landline telephone link which can be activated by the service user pressing a button worn as a wristband or pendant etc. This then triggers an alarm call via a base unit to the monitoring centre. The centre will know their details and the trained and skilled operators can offer support or help to organise the care they need.

The base unit is the part of the telecare system which is connected to the phone line, and receives signals from the pendant and any sensors. The base unit has two cables attached; one cable connects to the phone line and the other cable plugs into an electric socket. The pendant and any sensors or alerting devices are wirelessly connected and communicate with the base unit via radio signals; this can be used around the home and within a short distance away in the gardens of the home. The base unit contains a speaker and microphone which allows a conversation with the monitoring centre if the alarm button is pressed. The microphone is quite sensitive so the user can be some distance from the base unit, even in another room, and still be heard by the call centre staff.

Newer units have additional functions which enable the unit to be used for activity monitoring across a number of timed periods. They can play back user recorded voice messages, for example to prompt medication, food or fluids; and some have an 'I'm OK' function which when pressed alerts the monitoring centre that the person doesn't require a call.

The monitoring centre is staffed 24 hours a day, every day of the year. If the alarm button is pressed the staff at the centre will automatically know where the alarm call came from and can bring up the user's details on their screen. They will talk to the person to find out what the situation is, or whether they were just testing the system or pressed the button by accident.

Control centres are run by a range of organisations including local authorities, manufacturers, commercial firms, housing associations or charities. The centres are staffed 24 hours a day, 365 days a year and the staff are trained in dealing with emergencies and will contact appropriate people and services quickly. They have different ways of getting help if help is needed, or if the operator cannot get a reply they will arrange for someone to visit.

The centre will hold the details of a few local people such as neighbours and relatives who are also likely to be a key holder or know the code to a key safe fitted at the property which contains a key for the home. The centre will telephone one of these people if the alarm is raised. Some areas may offer a mobile warden service – then the centre will send out a member of staff to help sort out the problem. This service is not available in all areas and may cost more than the standard nominated responder service.

Community and telecare services work closely with local fire and rescue services (FRSs). In some areas the local FRS may act as a responder or even install telecare sensors. A home safety check is offered to all vulnerable households: see www.fireservice.co.uk/safety/hfsc. They will also be likely to link to local home improvement agencies supporting people to maintain and adapt properties to meet their changing needs. To find local services, visit: http://foundations. uk.com/about-home-improvement-agencies/

Some community alarm systems are sold via online sites and will just link a pendant or wrist-worn alarm alert to a monitoring system. This can be all that someone requires. However, it can limit future flexibility if at a later stage they wish to link telecare sensors, such as smoke or carbon monoxide alerts, fall detectors, epilepsy detectors or door alerts among others. There is a useful website that can help you understand the current range of sensors and how they work: www.independentforlonger.com/. A short video, at online resource https:// vimeo.com/58473260, relays the customer experience and a third is a virtual house which shows how different telecare sensors function around a typical home: www.tynetec.co.uk/new-to-telecare/3d-house

The case study (Example 4.1) is linked to managing bed exit and risks of falls, but other sensors could be added or substituted to provide an alert for epileptic seizure, door exit, incontinence etc.

EXAMPLE 4.1 Keeping a person who is at risk safe in their own home

Jane lived alone and had experienced a number of falls which resulted in numerous trips to hospital. She became anxious about living alone and what would happen if she fell and was not found for a long period. Her family started to discuss with her the possibility of her moving into a care home. But she wanted to stay at home and was referred to the local falls team. They supported her with exercise and transfer skills, helped review her home environment and raised her chair and bed to a more suitable height for her to transfer; they added rails to help her negotiate steps, stairs and the landing at home.

Her medication was reviewed and Jane was issued with an automatic pill dispenser which was filled with her medication each week and programmed to alert her at the appropriate time each day when her medication was due to be taken. If she did not dispense the medication the device would contact the monitoring centre, where staff in turn could prompt her, over the base unit speaker.

This dramatically improved her taking of medication on a regular basis. In the daytime she wore a fall detector which if she fell would alert the call centre that she needed help. At night she had a bed exit sensor fitted under her mattress which was programmed to turn on her bedside, hall and bathroom lights when she got out of bed. It was set to allow her 10 minutes to return to bed, and lights dimmed once she was back in bed and the unit reset itself. If she did not return to bed within the allotted time, the device alerted the monitoring centre team who could check that she was safe and coordinate a response if required.

Similar set-ups to Jane's are commonly used to support onsite family carers and allow them to sleep, reassured that they will be alerted at night if help is required.

Take a look at this website to see a range of approaches and helpful resources relating to falls detection and use of telecare: www.coventry.ac.uk/Documents/ HDTI/HDTI_Falls_One%20Page%20Flyer.pdf. There is a link to a free app which helps to identify common risks around the home and then advises on how to mitigate them: https://cele.coventry.ac.uk/fallcheck/

For families who share the same home there are a number of easy to set up and use standalone telecare systems which alert the onsite carers. These are designed to work straight out of the box and link the sensor to a pager carried by the carer. There are no monitoring centre costs to fund and for some people these are a practical and popular choice starting from under £100 ex VAT for a sensor and pager. See www.youtube.com/watch?v=aFBWiZX52pc

EXAMPLE 4.1   (continues) Avoiding dehydration and increased risk of urinary tract infection

Jane struggled to make hot drinks. Her dexterity was affected by arthritis and much as she liked to drink a cup of tea, the effort of boiling water and tipping her kettle discouraged her from making tea. She drank less and began to experience frequent urinary tract infections, sometimes requiring admission to hospital when she became confused and dehydrated. She also became more isolated, being less inclined to invite friends around for her traditional coffee mornings. Overall she felt less capable, more isolated and more vulnerable.

Her friends were concerned and her occupational therapist suggested that she use a kettle tipper; see www.livingmadeeasy.org.uk/kitchen%20and%20household/ teapot-and-kettle-tippers-2312-p/

This is a device which holds a kettle and allows it to be poured easily. She liked the idea but being very house proud found the design not to her taste and felt that it would identify her as a disabled person. She went to an electrical store looking for a lightweight kettle and found a number of fast boil one-cup kettles. (See the example at www.livingmadeeasy.org.uk/products.php?groupid=597) This swiftly heats and dispenses boiling water straight into the cup, only heating the water required from a reservoir and having an adjustable flow control to suit any size of cup.

She purchased the kettle and immediately was able to prepare hot drinks whenever she wanted. Her risk of dehydration diminished, and hospital admissions were no longer triggered. Her confidence grew and her friends visited regularly again once the coffee mornings were reinstated. The cost of the kettle was around £50 – a fraction of the cost of the community nursing and hospital treatment now avoided.

AT exists for safer walking too. Location is identified via GPS (a satellite-based global positioning system as used in car satnav systems) and will allow authorised people to find your location provided you carry the device. GPS devices can be a specific battery-powered device or built into a mobile phone and will enable authorised individuals, such as relatives or carers, to find out someone's location by logging onto the Internet from a computer. Some come with a subscription for a monitoring service; others can be managed via family and friends. If there are areas near home which could pose a risk, a geofence is created (map coordinates of a predefined area are stored in the unit) and if the person leaves this area with the unit, an alarm or alert is raised to the monitoring centre or family and friends.

EXAMPLE 4.2 GPS supporting safer walking

Harry loved walking. He had a long career as a postman and in retirement enjoyed walking around his community frequently meeting his many friends and acquaintances. His local knowledge of the neighbourhood had been exceptional but long familiar landmarks changed, with pubs becoming supermarkets and blocks of flats. This confused him and as he aged and developed the symptoms of early dementia he occasionally got lost. His family were concerned and sought support and a place at a day centre.

During his assessment it was suggested a building-based service could be restrictive and a GPS technology was explained. In Harry's case his family purchased a mobile phone with GPS function for around £120. This allowed a two-way conversation and had a simple SOS button which if Harry pressed would contact three people who were willing to respond. The phone texted the location (accurate within a few metres) where he was and they could look at this on Google maps etc. They could speak to him and offer support, guidance and reassurance if he was lost. If he was late home from a walk his family could text the device for coordinates or speak with him.

This worked well for Harry and his family. They supported his independence and gained reassurance of being able to check his location which allowed him to continue as part of his community. The exercise and stimulation of meeting familiar faces each day enhanced his well-being.

Activity monitoring systems

Understanding the abilities and dependencies of people with cognitive impairment can be difficult. Activity monitoring systems can be very helpful when considering how people living alone function in their own homes. Visitors, family members and carers will all affect how people function as will assessments via hospital or respite facilities.

Perceptions of risk and how people spend their time can be subjective, frequently based on assumptions and prejudices. Having objective information on what actually happens supports a personalised approach, builds on a person's abilities and helps target care and the proportionate use of technology to support independent living and manage and mitigate risks.

These systems can also support informal carers (i.e. family and friends) to understand changes in someone's routine, providing reassurance that people are still managing in their own homes. There is a growing number of portable, easy to use activity monitoring systems available. Typically they include a range of motion sensors which are fitted in rooms and external doors. A base unit with a GSM sim card gathers movement activity and displays this on a secure web page accessible to those with password access. The screens will show movement and door activity 24/7. Interpreting these charts will allow family and assessors to understand patterns of someone's behaviour, their areas of ability and where support might be required.

This can be very effective in supporting people in transition from one environment to another, coping with a loss like the death of partner and living alone. It can also assist in the evaluation of whether telecare or standalone technologies are effective in managing and mitigating risks.

EXAMPLE 4.3 Activity monitoring can keep someone safe at home

Linda lived alone. Her neighbours reported hearing her leave her house late at night, looking for her daughter. Her daughter lived locally and visited her mother every morning before work. Frequently she found her mother sitting in the lounge in her nightwear when she arrived.

An activity monitoring system was installed with Linda's agreement. It showed

Linda going to bed at a regular time but sometimes when she woke to use the bathroom she would not return to bed, would leave the house and return 30 minutes later and then sit in the lounge until morning came.

She already had a community alarm, and so a bed exit sensor and lighting system were installed. In addition, a linked door exit alert and a standalone memo minder were placed in the hall near to the front door. Immediately the bed exit and lighting system showed its effectiveness in guiding her to and from bed but occasionally Linda would approach the front door.

Her daughter had recorded a simple reassuring voice message which said, 'Mum, go back to bed; I will see you in the morning.' This played back to Linda as she got close to the door and the system showed her returning to bed. In the event of her staying out of bed for longer than 10 minutes or exiting the house, the call centre would be alerted and could respond with a voice prompt via the base unit.

The latest versions of these systems have additional functionality in exception reporting and can be programmed to send an alert to a carer or an assessor if, for example, someone has not been in the kitchen or bathroom by given times. This could be the first indication that a person has stopped preparing drinks or has reduced their need to use the toilet and may indicate the first signs of dehydration.

Other uses can show someone lying in bed for longer periods, which might indicate that they have a low mood or that people are not following activity patterns set by their therapist. Families can rent or purchase these kits for longer term use with prices ranging from under £8 per week.

Cost savings from telecare?

There are some good examples of how telecare can provide more efficient service provision. Any ageing population in any country will trigger social and economic challenges – with a higher proportion of people and more numbers with long-term medical conditions and physical disabilities. Telecare is vital to support people in their own homes and prevent avoidable pressures on the NHS and care systems.

EXAMPLE 4.4 Councils promoting technology to the wider public

The West Midlands ATHome website is raising awareness of the wide range of Assistive Technology available through case studies and video clips www.athome.uk.com.

The ARCHIE framework that defines quality in assistive living technology[4]

A user-centred approach to the design and delivery of AT must be adopted if it is to be willingly used by the general population in need of technological assistance or who could benefit from it. The ARCHIE framework captures anchored, realistic, continuously co-created, human, integrated and evaluated elements. The six principles are as follows:

1. Design and development should be ANCHORED in a shared understanding of what matters to the patient or client.
2. The technology solution and care package should be REALISTIC about the natural history of illness and the (often progressive) impairments it may bring.
3. Solutions should be CONTINUOUSLY CO-CREATED along with patients and carers, using practical reasoning and common sense.
4. HUMAN factors (personal relationships, social networks) will make or break a telehealth or telecare solution.
5. The service must be INTEGRATED by maximising human awareness, coordination and mobilisation of knowledge and expertise.
6. EVALUATION and monitoring are essential to inform system learning.

So we need more personalised care solutions for technology enabled care for individuals that take account of a person's physical and cognitive abilities and their personal or sociocultural situation. A person's care should be supported by technology and health and social care teams, rather than dominated by a technological package.

FAQs

Q1. Where can I find more information about AT options?

A. There are a number of very useful and accessible online resources which provide information on a range of solutions, including a supported guide to find suitable products for a task or activity:

    www.dlf.org.uk/factsheets/telecare
    www.athome.uk.com/
    www.tynetec.co.uk/independentforlonger
    http://asksara.dlf.org.uk/ run by the Disabled Living Foundation
    www.livingmadeeasy.org.uk/
    www.moreindependent.co.uk/news/what-is-telecare/
    www.atdementia.org.uk/
    www.hft.org.uk/Supporting-people/Our-services/Personalised-Technology/
-An-Introduction/
    The short film at www.athome.uk.com/testimonials-2/ shows people using

AT options including Telecare, GPS, digital reminders, memo minders and pill dispensers.

The Alzheimer's Society also produces a fact sheet on AT at www.alzheimers. org.uk/site/scripts/download_info.php?fileID=1779

Q2. Is there a list of community alarm and telecare providers?

A. The Telecare Services Association (TSA) website has a postcode search facility to link you to accredited members: www.telecare.org.uk/service-provider-directory

Q3. How much does AT cost and who pays?

A. The cost of community alarms, for example, varies depending on the provider and the level of service offered. Many charge around £3.50–4.00 per week. Telecare is frequently provided free on loan by the local authority social care team following an assessment. The recipient will still need to fund their community alarm and the cost of their landline rental. Always ensure that people are claiming any benefits that they are entitled to. The introduction of direct payments within health and care services offers new opportunities to develop more creative, flexible TECS for them to select.

Standalone technologies are increasingly available on the high street and through Internet stores. It is always worth getting advice on what products might help and then comparing prices before self-purchase as there can be a wide variation in costs between catalogues, shops and retail outlets. Frequently, devices are exempt from VAT.

Shops and sources of technology:

http://wm-adass.org.uk/wp-content/uploads/2014/04/Products-and-information-v21.pdf

www.bhta.net/find-a-member

www.athome.uk.com/useful-information/

References

1. DH. *With Respect to Old Age: long term care – rights and responsibilities.* The Royal Commission on Long Term Care. London: Stationery Office; 1999. Available at: www. dlf.org.uk/anarchyoropportunity
2. Carers UK. *Potential for Change: Transforming public awareness and demand for health and care technology.* London: Carers UK; 2013. Available at: www.carersuk.org/for-professionals/policy/policy-library?task=download&file=policy_file&id=199
3. Local Government Association. *Transforming Local Public Services: using technology and digital tools and approaches.* London: Local Government Association; 2014. Available at: www.local.gov.uk
4. Greenhalgh T, Procter R, Wherton J *et al.* What is quality in assisted living technology? The ARCHIE framework for effective telehealth and telecare services. *BMC Med.* 2015; **13**: 91. doi: 10.1186/s12916-015-0279-6.

Chapter 5

Telemedicine and video or Skype consultations: gaining benefits, minimising risks and barriers, and overcoming challenges

Marc Schmid

Telemedicine

Telemedicine and teleconsultation include 'the use of video conferencing facilities (or high-quality webcams) to enable remote consultations between patients and healthcare professionals, as well as peer to peer consultations between professionals'.[1]

EXAMPLE 5.1   Skin cancer diagnosis

Doncaster Clinical Commissioning Group (CCG) has worked with a mobile technology company to create the 4GEE service that focuses on skin cancer diagnoses. GPs can connect a microscope to their own smartphones to take a detailed picture of the suspect skin lesion and email this to the associated skin specialists. The dermatologist team sends back the diagnosis promptly – within an average 48 hours, saving an estimated £70 a patient who would otherwise have been referred to the hospital outpatient department for a face-to-face consultation. (http://ee.co.uk/business/large/why-ee/4gee-case-studies/NHSDoncaster)

There is no specific accepted definition of 'telemedicine' and how this differs from the term 'telehealth'. It is often assumed that telemedicine includes a diagnostic element – such as teledermatology where a diagnosis is suggested or confirmed remotely (maybe requiring subsequent biopsy etc.). This renders the application a 'medical device' which requires accreditation.

Video consultations underpin telemedicine as in Examples 5.2 and 5.3 which show how telemedicine can be applied for different patient groups, in varied health settings for a specific purpose, and the improved quality of delivery of care.

EXAMPLE 5.2   Using telemedicine for people with learning disabilities

Adam Hoare, managing director v-connect; Alasdair Morrison, social care team manager

Goal
The better outcomes for people with learning disabilities (BOLD) project was set up to explore whether better use of remote care technology could be used to improve health outcomes for people with learning disabilities (LD).

The v-connect service has provided ways of developing new models of care, using two-way video into the home for over seven years. Examples exist in primary care linking GPs to care homes, supporting patients with long-term conditions to remain at home and in social care settings via virtual visiting. The BOLD project aimed to combine user-centred design and service transformation to meet these challenges using technology enabled care services (TECS). The goal was to holistically reassess people with LD on high-cost care packages to use appropriate technologies to improve their outcomes.

Method
There were three major components:
1. Assessment – holistic view and appropriate response.
2. Care package review – fitting technology to the needs of the person with LD.
3. Process – implementation and understanding of how mainstreaming could be achieved.

Overcoming barriers
There was a range of cultural and systemic challenges to implementing the remote support. Overcoming these required a range of engagements and mitigations that included:

- case conferencing with family, advocates or support workers to explain what needed to happen, and how technology would support and protect service users

- service user visits to Sandwell Telecare Assisting You (STAY) offices to see how technologies work and understand how they would assist them with their day-to-day living
- allowing all to touch, feel, play with and use equipment in order to overcome barriers; embedding of trusted assessor training and telecare provision within social worker roles
- allowing simultaneous provision of existing support and technology with clear timetable for removal of support elements
- timely reviews and case conferencing to ensure that packages were complementary, allowing for identified reductions to be made.

Case reviews
Of the 60 cases reviewed, 33 people with LD were reassessed and considered appropriate for change as part of the project. Ten people had the video communication service installed as part of their care package. By connecting them to the community alarms provider they could have visual access to support 24 hours per day.

Financial impact
Total savings against budgets for the 33 cases over a period of 12 months was £515 000.

Taking the BOLD approach further
The early success of remote video support encouraged the exploration of how learning-disabled people would, themselves, like to be supported remotely. The user-centred design has been undertaken in collaboration with the care providers and with the local authority and CCG. The next stage is to develop technology specifically aimed at improving access to healthcare and promoting independence for people with LD.

Quotes
'I have been very surprised and you did prove me wrong. I know in the beginning I felt that you were putting these boys at risk; however, this technology has given them some independence back and allowed them to do tasks I felt they couldn't do. I am so proud of them both and I think it has been fantastic for them.' (Carer)

'I found the video very useful when I broke a glass in the kitchen; the lady told me what to do to clean it up and told me which bin to put the glass in as I was worried one of us would cut ourselves.' (Person with LD)

The project was delivered by v-connect for Sandwell Metropolitan Borough Council and funded by Health Enterprise East in collaboration with Yorkshire and Humber Academic Health Science Network through the Small Business Research Initiative (SBRI).

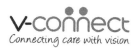

EXAMPLE 5.3 Telemedicine can underpin renal remote delivery of care

Adam Hoare, managing director, v-connect

Goal

The aim was to provide remote care as a holistic approach to support renal replacement therapy along the patient pathway. This would address the challenge for more renal care to be delivered closer to home via remote delivery that communicated with patients and monitored their physiological conditions. Many people who choose home dialysis (as opposed to hospital based) improve the normalisation of their daily lives and are less dominated by disease. They exhibit considerable self-management skills and do not perceive themselves as ill, but they still require close contact with hospital staff for communication and follow-up.

This project was initiated to introduce a renal telemedicine service for the management and support of service users on home haemodialysis, peritoneal dialysis and those with stable transplants. This enabled the hospital to place patients at the centre of their care and support them to be more empowered. The project was initially funded for six months.

Clinical delivery

The video communication service was deployed in 40 patients' homes. Clinical outcomes during the first six months included:

- replacement of 13 clinics with remote teleclinics
- more than 50 video consultations with patients at home
- introduction of ad hoc video calls into the renal department during clinic hours
- strong clinical engagement with five consultants using the video (two transplant and three nephrologist) and positive renal nurse engagement.

Technological achievements

The clinic successfully established the use of video in renal care and IT connectivity within the hospital. The service provided proof of concept for:

- weight and blood pressure measurements relayed back to the hospital during a video consultation
- dialysis data from a Fresenius home haemodialysis machine back to the database in the hospital
- interaction with the data card use by the peritoneal dialysis machine remotely in the patient's home
- high resolution images relayed back to the hospital for inspection of fistulae and technical issues
- integration of data storage with a database already in place in the hospital.

Outcomes

1. Patient and carer benefits:
   - avoided travel to and from hospital
   - reduced economic cost for family and carers (e.g. lost time off work)
   - increased patient confidence and reduced anxiety
   - immediacy of support
   - improved patient education
   - enhanced compliance and concordance with therapy or medication
   - family and carer engagement in care
   - logged savings of 84 hours and 3360 miles (5407 km) of patient travel during the six-month pilot project.

2. System benefits:
   - increased clinic efficiency
   - avoided hospital transport costs
   - increased nurse efficiency
   - increased consultant efficiency
   - reduced acute events such as A&E attendances and unplanned events
   - improved access to patient data including access to home dialysis data and high resolution images.

Patient quotes

- 'Why didn't they do it before?'
- 'Much more relaxed than clinic B.'
- 'The hospital transport always takes me round the villages and I don't get home for ages.'
- 'You feel as if the person is next to you talking to you – like now I am talking to you.'
- 'I would rather see a face in front of me and talk to them.'

This project was a collaboration between East and North Hertfordshire NHS Trust and v-connect funded by Devices for Dignity and the SBRI.

Video consultations are being increasingly applied for remote interactions between a patient and healthcare professional and between health and social care professionals.

In practice, the use of video technology may be as simple as two clinicians discussing a case via Skype or as complex as bespoke video technology linking GP practice teams with care homes such as is happening in Staffordshire. Increasingly, there is a need to explore the use of readily available platforms such as Skype or FaceTime which offer the potential for interacting directly with patients. This could be as part of a self-monitoring programme or an asthma review consultation.

Several large consulting firms have forecast that virtual physician visits will soon be the norm in the USA. Deloitte has reported that as many as one in six doctor 'visits' are already virtual. In many American cities you can even use a mobile app to request a doctor's house call.[1]

Care at a distance or 'in absentia' care has been running for years in different manifestations (*see* Example 5.4 on long-distance neurology services that were in place until 2004); but as technology develops the challenge is to radically change the way health services are delivered. As pressure builds from the bottom up, the system itself will be under pressure to meet the new 'digital native' patient who wants to email and Skype the nurse as well as monitor their own health through wearable technology. The introduction of video consultations is beginning to disrupt traditional care pathways. As homes and people become more connected and we see a growth in the *Internet of Things*, patients will expect the health system to be up to speed with their demands for flexible modes of delivery of care.

EXAMPLE 5.4   How a telemedicine service for Parkinson's disease operated more than 10 years ago (Dr Beatrice Summers, consultant neurologist, University Hospital, North Midlands)

'Until 2004, I ran a neurology service which had been set up using a webcam. I used to be responsible for neurological services in Cannock and Rugeley as well as Stafford. There was a cable between hospitals in Stafford and Cannock (which probably is no longer used as these hospitals are now owned by two different NHS trusts). A webcam was installed for my use in a clinic room in Cannock Hospital. I could look at the images from my computer in the Stafford Hospital.

'A receptionist would take an individual patient and usually a relation to the room at a designated time.

'Patients would travel from Tamworth as well as from local areas of Cannock and Rugeley. When they arrived, I would telephone them. I could see how well their Parkinson's disease was controlled.

'I used this system for alternate follow-up appointments. I had made the initial diagnosis on a face-to-face basis.

'I asked for feedback from the patient and their relation. The majority of individuals were happy with this service, though the odd individual felt it did not suit them. The service did not involve Skype. I was never able to extend my service so that local GP practices could be linked with my computer.

'These days telephone clinics are standard for Parkinson's disease, but they do not enable visual assessment of people's motor difficulties.'

According to a report from Tractica in the USA, the extent of telehealth video consultations across the globe is increasing.[2] Tractica forecasts that the market for devices, software, services and applications in this area will see strong growth over the 2014 to 2020 forecast period. Starting from a base of 19.7 million consultations in 2014, the market will expand at a compound annual growth rate (CAGR) of 34.7% through to 2020, by which time 158 million sessions are forecasted to be performed annually.

This presents the UK health and social care systems and others with a challenge. Are we in a position to be able to deliver this form of service delivery? And do we have enough knowledge within the system to ensure that services at the front line have the confidence to roll out the use of video consultations? Might patient or service user safety be at risk if video consultations are substituted for face-to-face care? Is the increased efficiency and productivity expected from Skype or video consultations worth the effort?

Benefits

As the Tractica research outlines, remote healthcare services and technology are quickly becoming commonplace across the globe. Telemedicine is enabling health professionals to evaluate, diagnose and treat patients remotely using the latest technology. In many situations, the use of video technology offers benefits as an alternative to traditional face-to-face support including the following:

- Minimising travel: many patients find it difficult to travel to hospitals, nurse clinics or GP practices for any number of reasons. The use of video can be a great option for patients where travel is difficult, as an option to traditional care. It can be particularly beneficial for those in isolated communities in rural parts of the UK where public transport access is limited or where travel to large cities may be a daunting prospect. A good example could be a weight management clinic with a high number of young mums on the register where childcare is an issue for them so Skype or FaceTime could help connect them to a health professional from the comfort of their home. In Lancashire, Skype was used in the urgent care service to connect deaf patients with interpreters. This reduced waiting times for the patient and costs to the hospital associated with callout fees.
- Improving networks: besides doctor-to-patient communication, video conferencing allows hospitals to create networks to provide each other with support. By easily sharing their expertise outside their own organisations, medical or nurse specialists can offer incredible value to their health or social care colleagues.
- Reducing the spread of infections: remote consultations can eliminate the possible transmission of infectious diseases between patients and medical staff. This is particularly an issue where spread of flu or MRSA is a concern.

- Reducing stress: the offer of a remote consultation via video link will not only relieve the pressure of the patient visiting the health practitioner, which can be daunting for some who suffer from 'white coat syndrome', but also ensures that those with phobias do seek medical help if required.
- Encouraging self-care: the use of video consultations can also be linked to self-monitoring equipment to ensure that patients or service users are using the equipment properly to take their readings.

Challenges to using Skype as a mode of delivery of care

Before you set up Skype you will need to consider a number of factors. Initially you should have discussions internally with IT providers and information governance (IG) services to ensure that they are comfortable with the approach. Example protocols which can be found on the website www.digitalhealthsot.nhs. uk have satisfied these types of concerns in CCGs and practices and include medical defence organisation considerations. *See* the Appendices to this chapter too. You might adopt or adapt some sections or a document for your own purpose – taking your own professional responsibility for the document that must fit with local IG and security procedures.

The second key aspect will be promoting the service and gaining consent from patients or service users. You will need to be clear with the patient that this form of consultation does not replace the existing services but enhances them. Patients will need to be selected to ensure that you are not adding to an already stretched workload. These patients may be ones who are responsible for repeat non-attendance or may be suffering from a long-term condition where accessing GP services is difficult. They may also be using self-monitoring equipment. Once you have agreed the approach you can begin the process of organising the Skype clinics. This is straightforward and involves the practice or clinic compiling the Skype contact list, messaging the patient to inform them when their consultation will take place and then contacting them at the given time as you would with a telephone consultation. It is important before commencing any consultation that you again ask the patient to confirm that they are happy using Skype and that they are broadcasting from a private room.

The equipment required is straightforward – a laptop or PC and webcam but you will need to check your broadband connection speed beforehand by testing the approach before going live.

Examples 5.5, 5.6, 5.7 and 5.8 all illustrate how different healthcare teams are using Skype to deliver care to their patients.

EXAMPLE 5.5   Pilot of 10 practices using different video consultation links to patients in own homes and local care homes

Stoke-on-Trent CCG is piloting the use of GP to patient interactions using video consultation via Skype. This project runs alongside a separate use of video technology (with v-connect) linking GP practices to care homes.

The use of Skype is seen as a low-cost but effective method of engaging with hard to reach patients or those who find it difficult to get to the practice and who may be prone to not attending or late cancellations. The project has involved enabling designated practice PCs to access Skype as well as training for staff to use it. A clear protocol is in place around the process of contacting the patient, and consent forms are distributed and signed beforehand. There are 10 practices on the pilot and each one is allowed to decide which patient group is best for them. Some examples include using Skype to link with patients with a long-term condition who are also using self-monitoring equipment. This allows the clinician to ensure the equipment is being used properly as well as ensuring the patient does not have to visit the practice. Other uses include weight management clinics for people with children who may find childcare an issue if they have to visit the practice as well as asthma reviews with teenage patients. Some practices are exploring using Skype to feed back test results for those patients who do not want to come into the practice but feel that the use of telephone is too impersonal.

All Skype–Skype voice, video or file transfers and instant message interactions are encrypted; but a call from Skype to a mobile or landline phone is not. Then the part of your call involving the ordinary phone network is not encrypted. Skype is on the NHS G-Cloud which contains approved software for use by NHS organisations.

EXAMPLE 5.6   Use of Skype underpinning sign language interpretation

East Lancashire Hospital Trust piloted the use of Skype in urgent care with deaf patients. The normal process for communicating with deaf patients who visited urgent care was to contact the local Deaf Society which would arrange for an interpreter to visit the hospital. This had a cost attached to it but also prolonged the length of time a patient had to stay in one of the UK's busiest urgent care units. The pilot project involved providing staff at the hospital with a laptop equipped with Skype that was directly linked to an iPad handed to the on-call interpreter. Staff in the urgent care team received training in the use of Skype and the laptop was stored securely near to the triage team. In the event of a deaf patient arriving at the urgent care department, hospital staff were able to contact the interpreter via Skype, reducing the on-call time as well as the length of patient's stay in urgent care. Posters were displayed in urgent care informing patients that the service was available.

EXAMPLE 5.7   Use of FaceTime

Seriously ill patients at Liverpool's specialist brain hospital the Walton Centre have been able to talk to their families using adapted Apple iPads.

The centre used the technology to allow patients silenced through illness to communicate with doctors and also loved ones at home using FaceTime video calls. The iPads were fitted on hospital trolleys. There are two on a trolley and the screens tilt over patients. One iPad points at the patient's face and the second shows the written messages, allowing relatives to see and communicate with their families.

Example 5.8 confirms that the majority of patients welcome Skype consultations as those with Parkinson's disease did in Example 5.4.

EXAMPLE 5.8   GPs pilot the use of Skype with patients

GPs at Cavendish Health Centre in London piloted the use of Skype consultations with patients, with 95% of patients involved saying they 'would use it again'.

Ninety-four per cent reported that they were satisfied or gave a better rating that the consultation had met their medical needs and 78% were satisfied with how long they waited for the appointment.

NHS Central London CCG found that a broad mix of patients had used the service including working people and parents of young children. Two-thirds of patients joined the remote consultations from home but more than a quarter – 28% – Skyped from their workplaces.

Dr Alice Fraser, the lead GP at the pilot practice, said: 'The flexibility that remote working offers means clinicians can make more efficient and productive use of time … Our patients with mobility or transport problems could get a more detailed consultation via Skype than a telephone conversation might allow, so this service proved especially useful for them.'

Risks and barriers

The downsides of using video technology include the cost of provision of the equipment and training for staff who will use it. Adopting a 'train the trainer' approach will encourage adoption by cascading learning throughout the organisation. Virtual consultations may also lead to potentially decreased interaction with the health or social care practitioner, so clear forward planning is required to determine the types of intervention where remote consultations will be used. This is also important to ensure that remote consultations don't become another additional pressure on the organisation.

Services that have used Skype for consultations often report that the use of video consultation focuses the patient on the issue for which they want help. However, for it to work effectively and be embedded within day-to-day practice, the use of video consultation has to show that it is reducing time, pressure and the cost of health or social care usage as well as improving the quality of service for the patient. This will allow clear business cases to be developed to roll out its use.

There is a school of thought that suggests virtual consultations can lead to overprescribing as the health practitioner errs on the side of caution. The setting of clear parameters for clinical protocols from the outset can address this.

A key barrier to adoption will be internal cultures within an organisation. Concerns about security will often be at the top of the list. When developing a case for use of video consultation, it is important to acknowledge that most interventions carry a risk. The use of postal services to carry information to a patient is not without risk. Telephone consultations or the use of email are not without risk either – where you cannot be absolutely sure that the recipient is the patient or service user you are meant to be communicating with. The key is about managing the risk at a level that your organisation feels comfortable with. Stoke-on-Trent CCG has developed a number of protocols and documents that will help organisations manage the risks. These have been endorsed by their Caldicott Guardian. The Standing Operating Procedure form for the rollout of Skype in general practice and associated Privacy Impact Assessment IG document can both be found on the website www.digitalhealthsot.nhs.uk alongside an example practice protocol, which is included (in brief) as Appendix 1 in this chapter. The best practice and checklist example from Nottingham included here as Appendix 2 should be helpful too.

FAQs

Q1. What are the barriers to implementing telemedicine?

A. Setting up telemedicine needs to happen at scale if it is to be effective – as in Example case studies 5.2 and 5.3. That requires planning, engagement and some upskilling with prior agreements on IG, privacy impact assessment, informed consent, medical defence organisation indemnity, protocols as well as the cost and set-up of equipment (maybe encrypted video link, or webcams) and upskilling (patient or service user, clinicians, administrators). But you can overcome these challenges by building on the learning from the various chapters of this book.

Another concern is about the security of Skype – and common FAQs are answered at: https://support.Skype.com/en/faq/FA31/does-Skype-use-encryption

Q2. How will the use of video consultation help reduce demand on health services?

A. There are some excellent examples of where the use of video is beginning to reduce demand on services. For example, in Roundwood Surgery, Forest Town, Mansfield they have created virtual ward rounds within a care home using iPads. The GP has a one-to-one consultation with their patient using Skype. Virtual ward rounds were completed between a GP from Roundwood Surgery in Mansfield and Stone Cross, a learning disability residential home. Prior to the introduction of the virtual ward if a client was ill, both transport and carers would be required to take them to the practice. This could be very disruptive for residents with severe LD. It also reduced the numbers of staff on duty within the home. The introduction of virtual ward rounds has allowed the staff at Stone Cross to spend more quality time with their clients. The GP has reported that holding regular virtual ward rounds has improved the levels of care delivered to residents and reduced demand.

Q3. How do you decide which form of telemedicine should be used?

A. This is entirely dependent on budgets and support from the IT teams. You may feel that the use of Skype or FaceTime is too risky for your organisation, which would lead you towards an encrypted system such as that provided by v-connect. If you are happy to adopt or adapt the protocols that are available with this book or perhaps don't have a budget to install bespoke equipment then low-cost options such as Skype and FaceTime have been tried and tested and are available.

Q4. What are the benefits of Skype/video consultations from a patient's perspective?

A. They:

- provide convenient and increased accessibility to your clinician (e.g. GP or practice nurse)
- enable you to discuss any health concerns or worries you might have
- give your clinician an opportunity to treat any health issues in a timely manner
- might help you to avoid visits to your GP practice or A&E.

References

1. Taylor K. *Connected Health: how digital technology is transforming health and social care*. London: Deloitte Centre for Health Solutions; 2015. Available at: www2.deloitte.com/content/dam/Deloitte/uk/Documents/life-sciences-health-care/deloitte-uk-connected-health-sm1.pdf
2. www.tractica.com/research/telehealth-video-consultations/

Appendix 1. Example practice protocol for Skype or video consultations with patients in their own home or a nursing/care home

Stage 1. Practice organisation and set-up

Practice manager or clinician affirms that medical defence organisation covers this activity.

It is the responsibility of the individual clinician to decide on the suitability of using Skype or video technology (as opposed to face-to-face consultation in surgery or patient's [care] home setting; or telephone or email consultation) per presenting complaint for each patient.

- *Nursing or care home:* The XX organisation will set up the video consultation equipment in each nursing or care home that has agreed to participate.
- *Individual independent patients:* Skype should be set up in one consulting room in the practice that is designated for Skype or video consultations (practice manager confirms which room), utilising a spare screen monitor if one available. If necessary your IT service provider should lift the firewall from practice computers once Privacy Impact Assessment/ Standard Operating Procedure documents are endorsed by CCG's Caldicott Guardian.
- *Skype security:* The practice needs to avoid people being able to search for doctors or practice nurses as individuals randomly without clinician invitation to a booked consultation. Go to 'tools', 'options' and then 'privacy'. This will also help practice to avoid falling prey to a phenomenon called 'vishing' (short for 'video phishing'). You can also block specific users in the 'options' menu.
- *Training:* Skype/video pilot lead supported by XX will upskill practice team including clinicians who will use Skype or video consultation technology. Training will include set-up, selection criteria, informed consent etc.; with appropriate paperwork (*see* Appendices 1.1 and 1.2).
- *Evaluation:* each clinician will capture information about the patient Skype or video consultation using data collection form for the first XX patients.

Stage 2. Prior to Skype or video consultation

2.1 *Patients might measure biometrics*

Prior to Skype or video consultation or during it – by arrangement: e.g. blood pressure, temperature, weight, oxygen saturation, pulse rate, blood glucose, sputum colour, peak flow. The clinician should ensure that any equipment used is valid and reliable, and the patient has been trained to take that measurement in reliable way (e.g. sphygmomanometer, peak flow meter).

2.2 *Inclusion and exclusion criteria proposed for patients who might consult remotely via Skype or encrypted video link between practice and nursing/care homes*

Practice team will trial these potential selection criteria for selecting patients to conduct remote consultations. After three months selection criteria will be modified to take account of clinicians' experiences. It is the responsibility of each clinician to select patients for Skype or video consultation depending on their symptoms, signs, cognition, support, confidence, preferences.

a. Skype – by GP or practice nurse with independent patient in own home or patient's chosen private setting

Inclusion criteria:

- children aged between 13 and 15 years with parental consent
- 16 years of age and above
- routine review by practice nurse or GP of any chronic condition, including:
  —asthma
  —diabetes (including follow-up for insulin initiation)
  —depression (mild/moderate)
  —anxiety (mild/moderate)
  —smoking cessation (follow-up)
  —hypertension review (with home blood pressure monitoring readings)
  —COPD review
  —epilepsy review
  —weight management.
- medication review
- low-risk patients requesting a consultation for any symptom (*see* following Stage 3).

Exclusion criteria:

- children aged 12 years and under
- acute deterioration of the above chronic conditions
- any condition requiring face-to-face clinical assessment or clinical examination
- intermediate- to high-risk patients for specific symptoms (*see* following Stage 3).

b. Encrypted video consultation – by GP or practice nurse with resident registered patients in nursing/care homes

Inclusion criteria:

- 16 years of age and above
- any chronic health condition for routine review including:
  —asthma
  —diabetes
  —depression (mild/moderate)
  —anxiety (mild/moderate)
  —smoking cessation (follow-up)
  —dementia (mild/moderate)
  —hypertension review (with home blood pressure monitoring readings)
  —COPD review
  —epilepsy review
  —lifestyle habit review.
- medication review
- intermediate- or high-risk patients judged to be reasonably well and alert, requiring a consultation for any symptom where there is an ability in the home for care home staff to assess and convey basic vital signs reliably, e.g. heart rate, temperature, oxygen saturation levels, blood pressure readings (*see* Stage 3 for further details)
- review of rashes
- urinary infection – proven by urine dipstick already.

Exclusion criteria:

- low- or intermediate-risk patients who care home staff feel are distinctly unwell (and for instance will need clinical assessment of heart and lungs)
- high-risk patients where it is not possible to monitor vital signs.

Distinguishing between high- and low-risk patients (risk is based on the potential significance of the presenting complaint given their past medical history or care home staff description of patient's symptoms)

Low risk	Intermediate risk	High risk
0–2 co-morbidities Co-morbidities that are present must be of low significance in terms of patient longevity, e.g. osteoarthritis (OA)	≥3 co-morbidities of any significance Co-morbidities present should not be directly related to presenting complaint	≥3 co-morbidities of any significance Co-morbidities that could be related to presenting complaint Current or previous diagnosis of cancer Age >90 years Poor mobility Dementia

Examples of each
Low risk:

- 20-year-old male, past history – eczema; complaining of slightly low mood
- 80-year-old female, past history – OA, hypertension; complaining of dysuria.

Intermediate risk:

- 50-year-old overweight male, past history – hypercholesterolaemia, hypertension (both well controlled); complaining of lower back ache
- 70-year-old female, past history – two transient ischaemic attacks (TIAs), hypertension, raised cholesterol; complaining of skin rash on lower legs.

High risk:

- 80-year-old female, past history – vascular dementia, COPD, hypertension; complaining of worsening breathlessness with a cough productive of clear sputum
- 90-year-old male, past history – ischaemic heart disease, two previous stent insertions; complaining of chest wall pain.

Stage 3. Conducting the Skype or video consultation
3.1 *Skype for patient who lives in own home*
The GP or practice nurse explains to the patient how the remote consultation will take place and gives them a copy of the information leaflet (*see* Appendix 1.1). If they want to proceed to plan a future Skype consultation the GP or practice nurse obtains written, informed consent at preceding face-to-face meeting (*see* Appendix 1.2).

Once the patient has given informed consent to use Skype they will need to give the clinician or practice staff their Skype ID details so they can add them to the list of Skype contacts the practice holds. To do this they search for the patient's name in the Skype search bar and then send them a request to be on the list of practice contacts. Add individual patient's details rather than wait for them to send the practice a request so you are sure they are the correct person. Advise the patient that they should set up Skype at their end in a private area and ensure that only people they are happy can overhear or view their Skype consultation are nearby.

Ask the patient to make a booked Skype consultation with specific clinician in reserved appointment slots or book in yourself. To make a Skype call ensure that you've got a webcam plugged in; click the green video call button to make it a Skype video call.

Useful things you can do on a video call:

- resize the screen – click and drag the corner of the video screen to make it bigger or smaller
- move it around – click and drag the video of yourself around your screen
- instant message (IM) at the same time – click the 'show messages' link at the top of the video to IM while you're on the call. If you are having any problems with Skype visit https://support.Skype.com/ where you can access more tips and ask questions.

If there is no Skype connection with the patient or they do not answer when the clinician initiates the Skype connection, clinician will leave a message (press the '+' symbol and click on 'video message').

The clinician should be clear from the start that they are allocating a fixed amount of time and that they will contact the patient, **NOT** the other way around – at a booked time. This will ensure that there is no expectation on the patient's part that they can use Skype for other issues. If a patient does contact the practice by Skype, simply decline the call.

3.2 *Video consultation between GP or practice nurse and staff or patients in a care/nursing home*

The practice guidance is similar to that for Skype usage described in 3.1. The practice clinician or nursing/care home staff can gain written informed consent from individual patients (so long as they can understand the process); if the patient is unable to understand the request for informed consent, the care home staff can do so on their behalf (in similar way to care home staff deciding when a patient requires a home visit from a GP).

The consulting area for video or Skype in the nursing or care home should be private – in a similar venue to that for a face-to-face consultation with GP. The room should be well lit so that the patient's image is clear.

If the Skype or video session is already connected and paused from a previous patient, a care home staff member will recommence the call and clarify that the next patient's privacy is assured (i.e. the previous patient has left the room). The care home staff will end the Skype or video consultations once all patients have been seen and discussions between GP or practice nurse and care home staff have been completed.

Stage 4. During the Skype or video consultation

Throughout the entirety of the consultation the following approach must be taken: usual best practice clinical management, careful active listening, frequent checking for understanding and an interested response.

If during the Skype or video consultation it transpires that a face-to-face consultation should take place, this should be arranged in an appropriate timeframe.

The clinician should write up notes of the consultation in the usual way in the patient's medical records. They should not make a video recording of the consultation, unless they're prepared to gain further specific informed patient consent and adhere to the detailed national information guidance and confidentiality requirements.

Remote consultation checklist for clinician or practice team

		Practice staff* or clinician** action
1.	The patient*** has received an explanation of the use of Skype/video for a remote consultation with the clinician	Practice staff – any
2.	A copy of the remote consultation patient information leaflet has been given and explained to the patient	Practice staff – any
3.	Any concerns about remote consultation have been addressed	Clinician
4.	The remote consultation patient consent form has been given and explained to the patient	Clinician
5.	The remote consultation consent form has been signed by the patient or their representative	Clinician
6.	The clinician has prepared his/her consulting room to maximise privacy	Clinician
7.	The patient is undertaking the consultation from their home or chosen private setting (or care home) at pre-agreed time booked into specific clinician's appointment list	Patient (and care home staff)
8.	The Skype call is instigated by the clinician at a date/time which has been agreed with the patient (or care home staff). Clinician logs onto Skype system and searches for patient Skype ID and then clicks the video call button	Practice staff – any
9.	On answering the Skype call, the patient should acknowledge whether or not it is appropriate to undertake the consultation	Patient
10.	The clinician will introduce themselves to the patient and: • confirm that the patient is happy to take part in the remote consultation, making it clear that if a physical examination is required, the clinician will invite the patient to come to the practice (or visit the Care Home if appropriate, i.e. patient housebound) • the patient's identity should be checked by asking them to confirm their name and date of birth	Clinician
11.	Prior to concluding the consultation, the clinician will clarify that the patient understands the outcome of the consultation and has no further questions	Clinician
12.	The clinician will record the bodily measurements that patient provides, observations and outcomes of the consultation in the same way as a face-to-face consultation is recorded in the patient's electronic primary care record and any agreed actions are carried out	Clinician

* Practice staff = any member of the practice team including administrator, receptionist, manager or clinician by arrangement.

** Clinician is the GP or practice nurse initiating and conducting the Skype/video consultation.

*** The term 'patient' used here means patient participating in Skype/video consultation or their carer/family.

Appendix 1.1. GP/nurse-directed remote consultations: patient information leaflet

Why are remote consultations being introduced?

To provide you with more regular access to your GP or practice nurse so that you can talk about any non-urgent health concerns or questions or also to make it easier for people to attend virtual asthma clinics to discuss their asthma and general health.

What is a remote consultation?

It is a conversation that happens between you and your GP or nurse – you can see and hear each other without being in the same room or building. It uses a technology called 'Skype' to allow you to see and hear each other. Lots of people use it all over the world to talk to family and friends who do not live near each other, for example in other countries.

What is Skype?

Skype is the programme that allows you and your GP or nurse to be able to hear and see each other. It works over the Internet.

Is Skype safe and secure?

Skype has been used in many other healthcare organisations with patients and there have not been any reports of security breaches. As with all information transmitted across the Internet, the security of Skype isn't 100%, but it is more secure than sending an email or posting a letter, so we believe the benefits outweigh the risks.

What happens if I don't want to talk to my GP or nurse in this way?

If you do not like this method of communication it can be stopped at any time. It is your choice whether or not you use it and we will answer any questions you may have before it is used and ask you for your written consent.

How will I be prepared for my remote consultation?

We will arrange to contact you at your Skype address at a set time which will have been arranged between you and the practice staff. When the GP or nurse starts the consultation with you, he/she will introduce themselves, check that you are happy to proceed and check your name and date of birth. At the end of the consultation they will check that you have understood the conversation and ask if you have any questions. After the Skype consultation has finished, the GP or nurse will write or type the outcome of the consultation in your medical record as usual.

What are the benefits of Skype or video consultations?

- They provide convenient and increased accessibility to your clinician (e.g. GP or practice nurse).
- They enable you to discuss any health concerns or worries you might have.
- They give your clinician an opportunity to treat any health issues in a timely manner.
- They reduce avoidable visits to the surgery or A&E.

What are the potential risks of Skype or video consultations?

There are potential risks associated with the use of Skype/video, but these are very small and the benefits of using Skype/video have been assessed as outweighing the risks. These risks include, but may not be limited to:

- information transmitted may not be sufficient (e.g. poor quality of video) to allow for an appropriate medical decision to be made by the clinician. In the event of this, a face-to-face visit with the clinician will be arranged
- although highly unlikely, security can fail, causing a breach of privacy of confidential medical information.

Appendix 1.2. Patient informed consent for Skype or video consultation

Practice

Patients under the care of XX practice can access a clinician via a Skype or video remote consultation. The remote consultation will provide you with the opportunity to speak to, and see, your clinician and have your health needs assessed on a remote basis; to discuss any existing health issues and other matters that you want to discuss. The Skype or video consultation is set up to meet national recommended standards to ensure data privacy for you as an individual patient.

My rights

- I understand that the NHS privacy and confidentiality policies and procedures relating to my medical information also apply to Skype or video remote consultations.
- I understand that the Skype or video technology used by the clinician is encrypted to prevent the unauthorised and unlawful access to my personal confidential data.
- I have the right to withdraw my consent to the use of Skype or video (opt out) at any time.
- I understand that the clinician has the right to withdraw (opt out) his or her consent for the use of Skype or video consultation at any time.
- I understand that the remote consultation will **not** be recorded.
- I understand that the clinician will not allow any other individual who is

not directly involved in my care to listen to, or watch, my Skype or video session.

Patient consent to the use of Skype or video for remote consultation

- I have read and understand the patient information provided regarding Skype or video. I have had the opportunity to discuss this information and all my questions have been answered to my satisfaction.
- I hereby give my explicit consent for the use of Skype or video in my medical care and authorise the clinician to use Skype or video to undertake remote consultations.

Patient name:	
Date of birth:	
Address:	
Patient's Skype identity details:	
Signature:	
Date:	

In the case of the patient not being able to give consent, the patient's name and address should be completed above in addition to the section below:

Name of patient's representative (e.g. carer/family, care home staff member):	
Capacity of representation (e.g. lasting power of attorney for their health and welfare; parent of child under 16 years of age; responsible care home staff member):	
Representative's address:	
Home's Skype identity details:	
Representative's signature:	
Date:	

Appendix 2. Records and Information Group Best Practice Guide for Nottinghamshire, Nottingham City Health and care services providers

Jayne Birch-Jones

Title: Teleconsultation guidance: best practice and checklist	
Date of Issue: XXX	Guide No.: YYY
Approved by: Records and Information Group [RIG]	Approved date: TBC
Replaces/Supersedes Guide No.: None	Distribution: All organisations (members of the RIG)

Scope:

All Nottinghamshire, Nottingham City Health and Care Services who wish to use video conference technologies to carry out patient or citizen remote consultations.

Evidence was collated and reviewed from a number of organisations that had deployed video conference technology to support consultations. This evidence was considered along with advice and guidance from the following bodies:

- Medical Defence Union
- Information Commissioners Office
- British Medical Association
- Royal College of General Practitioners
- Health and Social Care Information Centre
- NHS England.

In reviewing this body of knowledge and consulting with organisations across Nottinghamshire who are using these technologies the following guidance has been produced. The content of this guidance note should form the basis of a checklist of items to address as part of any service deployment.

1. Information Governance:

   a. Any deployment of a new way of working or change in process which involves the processing of personal and sensitive data must be approved by your organisation's Information Governance manager.

   b. A Privacy Impact Assessment must be carried out as part of the implementation of this way of working for every service.

   c. The patient or citizen should receive appropriate information relating to the consultation and associated risks to allow them to make an informed decision on consent to use the technology for this purpose (stakeholder engagement).

   d. Any information should be in a suitable format for the specific group of patients or citizens, e.g. large print might be considered for some groups of patients in nursing home care. Reference can be made to NHS England's accessible information standard.

   e. In making a decision in relation to consent there should be a consideration of patient or citizen capacity in line with professional assessment standards, organisational policies on consent and assessing capacity and the Mental Capacity Act 2005 requirements.

   f. When organising the consultation, consideration must be given to the environment in which it takes place. This should be secure, confidential and accommodate any special requirements the patient or citizen or care professional might have, such as: good lighting, appropriate space and comfort in the surroundings. You should also ensure that you maintain the patient's or citizen's privacy and dignity at all times.

 g. The appropriateness of all consultations should be risk assessed in line with recommendations for current practice in carrying out telephone consultations.

 h. As part of the agreement with the patient or citizen they must be made aware of potential risks relating to the consultation, e.g. any technical considerations when using public networks or non-corporate use of equipment at the patient or citizen end.

 i. It should be noted that the relevant Information Governance Toolkit requirements and standards apply similarly to use of any other equipment and should be adhered to.

2. Information Security

 a. Prior to any live service commencement (and as part of the Privacy Impact Assessment process) there must be Caldicott Guardian and Senior Information Risk Owner sign-off (or equivalent organisation governance for approval).

 b. Recording of consultations is generally not advised. If recording is requested by the patient it is essential that additional advice is sought on the management and storage of the recorded files. The patient would be obliged to agree that recordings, the patient end, should only be for personal or domestic use and further distribution could infringe the privacy rights of staff members without their consent.

 c. As part of the service deployment, all IT equipment used should be considered for suitability, including appropriate end point security and protection. All IT equipment used should be organisation owned, have appropriate encryption and virus software installed and included on the asset register. Use of personal equipment is prohibited.

 d. When selecting a video conference tool or solution the following requirements must be appropriately met:

  i. No residual data must be left on IT equipment.

  ii. Encryption standards must conform to the HSCIC [Health and Social Care Information Centre] requirements (http://systems.hscic.gov.uk/infogov/security/encryptionguide.pdf) which is currently 256 AES.

  iii. An independent security software assessment should be in place for any video conference software used that validates it has appropriate encryption, meets the organisation's system level security policy, appropriate key management, identity management and appropriate technology to prevent 'man in the middle' attacks.

  iv. Where consultations are intra-organisation, there should be internal administrative functions to support strong management of user policy.

  v. Where consultations are extra-organisation, steps should be taken to ensure user policy is applied wherever possible.

  vi. Apart from consultations that take place with the patient or citizen directly in their own environment, all kit should be corporately owned, managed or configured.

  vii. It is advised that as part of the organisation's annual risk assessments this should include use of new and evolving technologies such as teleconsultations; this could include penetration testing.

 e. It should be noted that the relevant Information Governance Toolkit requirements particularly in the 300 series apply and should be adhered to.

3. Custom and practice (Standard Operating Procedures)
a. When deploying video conferencing technology to support consultations a Standard Operating Procedure should be developed to ensure that users are clear on the process and appropriate assessment stages. Staff should be provided with the appropriate equipment training, where necessary, and in all circumstances ensure that they complete and remain in date with Information Governance training at all times.
b. Staff must ensure that they are aware and comply with organisational Information Governance and Information Security policies.
c. In line with professional body recommendations, records management processes must be in place to ensure contemporaneous and contiguous records are kept. Advice on this aspect is available from the relevant professional bodies. It is advisable for the organisation to amend its Records Management policy to reflect this change in the way of working.

Review date: XXX	File location:

Chapter 6

Apps: the future is mobile

Marc Schmid

'mHealth' can be defined as 'health-related mobile applications (apps) and health-related wearable devices'.[1] There are more than 165 000 health apps available in Europe, including those designed to support general health and well-being, those that help to monitor health conditions, apps for clinicians or carers and apps that function as medical devices.[2] Uses for personal wellness and activity tend to be initiated by individual consumers so there is less need for confidentiality of the data generated. When used for reporting to clinicians or patient/hospital systems, data confidentiality must be preserved.[1]

All apps in the UK are regulated by the Data Protection Act 1998 (DPA) and the European Directive on Misleading Advertising.[2] If an app is considered to be a medical device (i.e. it is used for diagnosis, prevention, monitoring, treatment; or alleviation of disease, injury or handicap; or investigating, replacing or modifying the anatomy or physiological process or controlling conception), it is regulated by the Medicines and Healthcare Products Regulatory Agency (MHRA) and required to attain a CE certificate.[3] If an app is not a medical advice, it may be added to the NHS Choices Health Apps Library (currently being updated) if it is thought to be relevant to people living in England, clinically safe and compliant with the DPA, with trusted sources of information such as NHS Choices. National consideration of what other regulation or endorsement is required for patient-focused healthcare apps in future is under way to find a method of evaluating a new app that is quick, robust and proportionate. There are particular concerns about compliance with data protection principles, and reliability of the content of the resources. So clinicians are advised that they should not use or recommend medical apps, including website apps, that do not have a CE mark; and clinicians should always exercise their professional judgement before relying on information from an app.[4]

Mobile medical apps are a prominent part of modern health and social care. The use of mobile medical apps by clinicians and members of the public has grown dramatically since the introduction of mobile phones and tablets. Mobile devices and apps can support a variety of routine medical tasks from viewing X-ray results to tracking symptoms and vital statistics. These apps help clinicians to diagnose, monitor and treat many common diseases such as drug dose calculation, patient education, accessing medical records, and clinical decision support. Medical apps offer clinicians the ability to access medical knowledge and patient data at the point of care with ease.

You can visit sites of interest by scanning the QR code with your smartphone or using the website address.

ORCHA SITE

ORCHA, the Organisation for the Review of Care and Health Applications, offers a platform of validated apps so the public and professionals have the confidence to use and recommend apps to revolutionise wellbeing and resources. Their platform aims to allow professionals, patients and the public embrace apps and at the same time have some reassurance that they are of sufficient quality and relevance.

As of publication the NHS apps library was under review.

www.orcha.co.uk

MY HEALTH APPS

My Health Apps brings together healthcare apps – tested and reviewed by patients and service users looking at changes in confidence, common problems and needs, achievements of targets or goals; trialled by Kirklees Council for promoting self-care and providing support for people with long-term conditions.

http://myhealthapps.net/category#

App stores now feature collections of apps dedicated to supporting healthcare professionals such as the Mersey Burns app (*see* FAQ 2, p. 104). The Health Apps Library provides some quality assurance to the apps listed by ensuring that they are reviewed by a panel of experts before being included.

The AliveCor mobile ECG is already being used in conjunction with a patient's own Android or iOS smartphone or device to record ECG. It can indicate atrial fibrillation and readings can be shared in real time with cardiologists in acute healthcare settings to help with interpretation and on the spot timely management. Other apps are being developed to examine all aspects of the eye, throat, mouth, lungs and throat.

The personal fitness app market has seen huge growth, supported by the development of wearable technology such as the Apple Watch and Garmin Vivosmart. However, in its report *mHealth App Developer Economics*[5] predicts that fitness apps, which today constitute the app category offering the highest business potential for mHealth app publishers, will reduce in importance and in five years' time no longer be in the top app category in terms of business potential for developers. The app categories that have the highest expected market potential in the near future are remote monitoring (53%) and consultation apps (38%). The mHealth apps are likely to have the biggest impact on healthcare system costs in two areas: reducing non-compliance with medication and other interventions, and minimising hospital readmission costs. There is a good case study in Example 6.1.

The Digital Health and Care Alliance has produced some helpful guidance on medical apps. You can access the document through this link: http://dhaca.org. uk/wp-content/uploads/2014/11/DHACA-Medical-Apps-Process-Document-interim-final.pdf

---

EXAMPLE 6.1   Wearable diagnostic device that can improve management of COPD to prevent avoidable deterioration

This wearable diagnostic device for chronically ill patients bridges the gap between personal and professional uses. Using a digital biosensor, the app can record biometric data of people suffering from chronic obstructive pulmonary disease (COPD), then relay that data to their HealthSuite digital platform using the patient's mobile device. This connects to an existing sensor, the HealthPatch, a cloud-based service that allows both patients and doctors an unprecedented level of access to real-time, round-the-clock health data.

Physical activity and inactivity, respiratory function, heart rhythm and heart rate variability are all monitored. The data is then retrievable via two apps, Philips eCareCompanion and eCareCoordinator, making it possible for doctors to monitor patients remotely. The HealthSuite digital platform should allow both patients and doctors to gain greater insight into patient health with more and better data presented in a user-friendly app. See www.usa.philips.com/healthcare-innovation/about-health-suite

---

According to figures from eMarketer[6] the number of smartphone users worldwide

will surpass 2 billion in 2016, representing over a quarter of the global population. That number is expected to grow to more than 2.56 billion people, or a
third of the world's population, in 2018 – by which time smartphones will finally
have overtaken feature phones in the telecommunications world. Ofcom's 2015
Communications Market Report found that a third (33%) of Internet users see
their smartphone as the most important device for going online, compared to
30% who are still sticking with their laptop. Smartphones have become the hub
of people's daily lives and are now in the pockets of two-thirds (66%) of UK
adults, up from 39% in 2012. The vast majority (90%) of 16–24 year olds own
one; but 55–64 year olds are also joining the smartphone revolution, with ownership in this age group having more than doubled since 2012, from 19% to 50%.
More details of the report can be found here: http://stakeholders.ofcom.org.uk/
market-data-research/market-data/communications-market-reports/cmr15/uk/
    This data is supported by the Deloitte Centre for Health Solutions which
reports that smartphone penetration in the UK is increasing in older people.[7]
The centre suggests that the baby boomers (born 1946–1964) generated the
fastest year on year growth in smartphone penetration in 2014.

How will increased use of apps transform health and social care?

Better access

In the modern digital age, a patient and their doctor need not be in the same
location. Patients suffering from long-term conditions who struggle to travel
either physically or financially can now access huge amounts of information
through mobile apps. In addition to this, apps such as Babylon or Push Doctor
offer people the opportunity to speak to a doctor via their smartphone for a
modest fee, and they can even be prescribed medication to be collected at local
pharmacies via the app. Instead of having the health system dictate that a visit
must be in person, patients and physicians can decide together when a visit is
best done live and when healthcare services can be delivered virtually.

Improved communication

The quality of communication between the health or social care system and
the patient is often criticised – sometimes rightly. Barriers are often placed in
the way due to internal processes or concerns around data security or quality.
Much of this is unnecessary. Technology is now available to speed up the system
and ensure that information is relayed to the patient or service user through the
channels which best suit their needs at a time they require it. People can now
be notified via their smartphones about the services they are accessing.

Encouraging self-care

Apps can now provide the patient with quality-assured information relating to
their health which can help them to manage it themselves. The vast array of

personal health information that is now captured by smartphone apps can be used by the patient to gain a better understanding of when they are well and when they need to see a doctor. According to a report from UK telemedicine company Push Doctor,[8] 23% of patients use a smartphone, tablet or computer to monitor exercise levels, 17% use such a device to establish their body mass index (BMI), 17% measure their heart rate, 15% establish daily diet and calorie intake, 13% monitor sleep quality and 5% share symptoms on social media to solicit friends' opinions. Although not providing medical grade data on the patient, this information can be used by the person to make personal decisions about their diet and lifestyle habits, which in turn can improve their health and well-being.

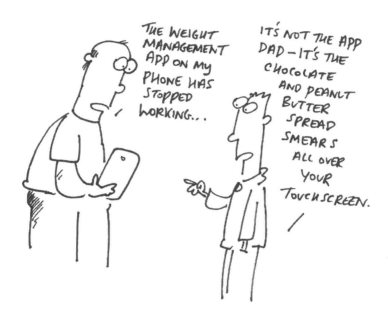

When leaving hospital or their GP practice, patients often have very little memory of the advice they were given about their condition and what to do next. Many will often search for advice on the Internet, which can be a dangerous place when it comes to health advice. Push Doctor analysed data[8] from over 61 million internet searches carried out in a 12-month period, looking at 160 of the most common health enquiries. In the 2014–15 year the number of health searches carried out in the UK increased by 19%, an increase of an average 848 820 searches each month. Table 6.1 produced by Push Doctor lists the most common health searches.

Apps that help to remind the person about what they need to do can help them to manage their illness and at the same time prevent them from having to seek further medical advice or access unverified medical advice from the Internet. Apps can be used to monitor medication usage to ensure that the person doesn't forget to take it or, as in the iVacc app, can store a record of a family's vaccinations and even send reminders when they are due.

TABLE 6.1 UK Health Search Index most common health searches

1	Back pain	100
2	Diarrhoea	94
3	Depression	89
4	Rheumatism	85
5	Multiple sclerosis	79
6	Meningitis	78
7	Chlamydia	72
8	Ovulation	63
9	Lupus	62
10	Diabetes	62
Index: most common search = 100		

Source: www.pushdoctor.co.uk/Resources/PushDoctor-Health-report.pdf

Apps that relay evidence-based recommendations about health conditions or lifestyle habits can enhance the quality of self-care that someone adopts – *see* the good case study in Example 6.2 of the UpToDate app.

EXAMPLE 6.2 UpToDate (www.uptodate.com/home/product)

This app offers evidence-based opinion and treatment recommendations on over 10 000 conditions (for a substantive cost). The information that goes into the app is peer-reviewed and collated by over 5000 doctors and clinicians.

The idea behind UpToDate is to come up with the types of questions that clinicians have when they're seeing patients, summarise the literature that can answer those questions and put that all together and provide recommendations for clinicians so they can not only answer those questions but can actually apply them to the users of the app. In the UK, about 100 hospitals subscribe to UpToDate, three-quarters of which are NHS trusts. A further 1700 individual doctors also subscribe to the service, which is accessible on desktop, iOS, Android and Windows Phone 8.

Doctors can also use UpToDate to reassure patients about their recommended treatment and give links to patient information sheets. This is a useful tool in the doctor–patient relationship.

Royal Liverpool and Broadgreen University Hospitals NHS Trust enables clinicians to use the app on their smartphones. This allows them to access up-to-date information for their own and for patients' education in a matter of seconds, rather than disrupting consultations. The trust delivers acute care services from two sites: Royal Liverpool University Hospital and Broadgreen Hospital, with a new hospital expected to be completed in 2017. With over 40 wards and more than 750 beds serving more than 465 000 people in Liverpool, the trust is a well-respected and innovative centre for patient care. See www.royalliverpoolacademy.nhs.uk/news/academy-award-winning-app

---

Enhancing provision of care

In the future, aspects of health and social care that can be provided digitally will be delivered remotely. Digital health apps will schedule appointments, help to monitor medications' side effects and help people to manage their own health. These changes will engage patients or service users with their healthcare in new ways as well as radically reforming health and social care delivery. The case study of Rally Round is a good example of this approach.

EXAMPLE 6.3   Rally Round

Rally Round is a website and mobile app developed by the Staffordshire-based company Health2Works. Developed in partnership with the NHS and local authorities, the app supports care networks by allowing them to manage a person's care in a secure environment. The person who needs care receives support via their immediate network which might consist of friends and relatives or professional carers. They can organise the care through the online platform which can include general household activities or other tasks such as to sort the weekly shop or take the person out for the day.

By managing the care in a simple way and ensuring that each person in the care network is notified when tasks have been completed or are outstanding, the use of the Rally Round app reduces the burden placed on certain family members to do all the tasks. Licences are purchased by health or social care organisations and integrated into their care programme so that carers are able to use the platform free of charge. See www.rallyroundme.com/welcome

---

There are online services being set up to provide a person with access to a GP in their area between 8 a.m. and 11 p.m. A patient can book a visiting doctor for any location of their choice – at their home, a hotel, an office, a holiday location. The associated app enables the linked GPs to turn their availability on or off. See www.gpdq.co.uk

Risks of apps

In the report 'mHealth and mobile medical apps: a framework to assess risk and promote safer use', the researchers examined some of the risks associated with health apps.[9] They described published evidence where some medical apps had compromised patient safety, being potentially dangerous for clinical use. These included some apps designed for opioid dosage conversion or melanoma detection, which they indicated demonstrate dangerously poor accuracy. They noted that many app developers have little or no formal medical training and do not involve clinicians in the development process; they may therefore be unaware of patient safety issues raised by inappropriate app content or functioning. There are so many medical apps that it seems impossible to assess each and every one. The report captured in Table 6.2 describes the different types of risks to which medical apps can contribute.

TABLE 6.2 Different types of risk associated with medical use of apps and scenarios where these may arise[9]

Type of risk in increasing order of severity	Main stakeholder affected	Sample scenario where this risk could arise	What can be done to manage this risk
Loss of reputation	Professional organisation	App displays sensitive performance data about professional or service	Good security
Loss of privacy, patient confidentiality	Patient	Poor security of patient data Lose phone holding patient data	Encryption Avoid holding patient data on mobile device
Poor-quality patient data	Patient, professional or organisation (e.g. financial data)	App allows bad data to be entered into patient record or retrieved from it at handover	Data validation on entry and retrieval from authenticated source
Poor lifestyle or clinical decision	Patient or professional	Bad patient data used in risk calculation algorithm Bad knowledge or search tool Bad advice or algorithm Poor risk communication	Check correct data retrieved Check algorithm properly coded Use proven health behaviour change methods
Inappropriate but reversible clinical action	Patient or professional	Poor medication advice	Test quality of advice on sample data Provide facility for user feedback and respond to this
Inappropriate and irreversible clinical action	Patient, professional or organisation (liability exposure)	Bad algorithm controlling insulin pump, surgical robot, radiotherapy machine etc.	Adopt safety critical software design and development methods Exhaustively check design and test algorithm and user interface

While welcoming the use of high-quality apps by health and social care professionals and patients or service users, the authors of the report argue that these risks give a significant chance of harm, and need to be mitigated. Care professionals should be educated about the risks posed.

Some people argue that healthy people shouldn't use health apps that monitor physical parameters because their readings are full of uncertainties, there's insufficient evidence of benefit or they might create unnecessary anxiety in a 'worried well' generation which might trigger many avoidable consultations with health professionals. Health practitioners will then need to become more competent at setting thresholds for when it is reasonable to worry about occasional cardiac arrhythmias for example, so that people who are reasonably healthy are not over-investigated or overdiagnosed or overtreated.[10] So health professionals should advocate health apps which encourage healthy behaviours that protect people's health and well-being, but be cautious about recommending apps that monitor people's physical function unless that is part of an agreed shared management plan.

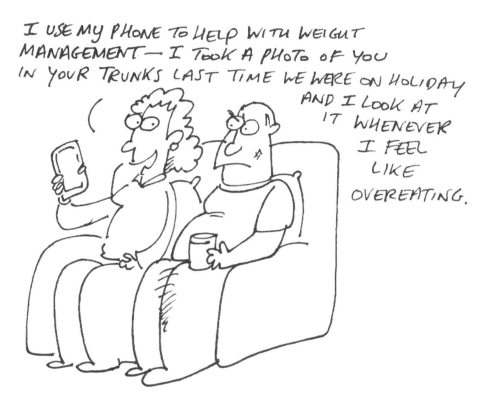

Improving access to services with an app

An app might be the technology to choose to improve access to services – as in the case study in Example 6.4.

EXAMPLE 6.4 Saving costs by a mobile application service

The London Borough of Lewisham's web and mobile app LoveLewisham enables local residents to report environmental issues. This has led to a 73% reduction in graffiti and 33% drop in call centre activity, saving £500 000 over a 5-year period.[11]

Example 6.5 describes an app that enhances access to urgent care for someone with an uncontrolled seizure.

EXAMPLE 6.5   Underpinning appropriate access to urgent care

Neutun's app uses a smartwatch's accelerometer to detect the shaking that signals epileptic seizures. If the watch registers that a seizure is happening, the wearer is asked to respond to an on-screen prompt. If no answer is received within a few seconds, notifications are sent to preset contacts and the watch displays relevant health information for emergency responders.

More usually an app may help someone understand and engage with treatment for their well-being (*see* Example 6.6) or their own long-term health condition (Example 6.7).

EXAMPLE 6.6   RoboCoaches help older people with their mobility

An android life-sized robot used in Singapore directs exercise classes for older people, using motion sensors to determine if they are doing the movements correctly. See www.digitaltrends.com/cool-tech/robocoach-helps-singapore-seniors-stay-in-shape/

EXAMPLE 6.7   Manage Your Health app

The School of Pharmacy at Keele University has developed an 'app framework' to support the delivery of healthcare messages for people with long-term conditions. Additional programming can be deployed to create a separate app for users to download. Clinicians evolve, check and sign off content. As well as useful health information and a personal log and diary, the app uses an innovative avatar to visually demonstrate health information and advice.

The app can relay updates to users and deliver a rich range of interactive materials on Apple or Android smartphones or tablets. Materials include text, images, interactive quizzes and activities with a 3D avatar giving information relevant to long-term conditions that users of the app may download. The app also uses augmented reality (AR) for patients with an Android or Apple smartphone or tablet with a built-in camera. The AR content will overlay information on top of the medication (e.g. an inhaler) to illustrate how best to use the medication; for example, demonstrating good inhaler technique and answering common questions to help the patient's own asthma management, via an avatar.

Generic content helps guide users towards a healthier lifestyle, covering topics such as managing stress, goal setting, exercise, healthy eating, managing alcohol consumption, quitting smoking, coping with financial concerns etc.

Visit Google Play Store at https://goo.gl/n1WswP or the Apple App Store at https://appsto.re/gb/nNL-9.i

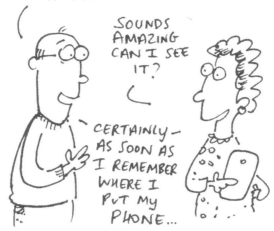

FAQs

Q1. Can you recommend a community app and describe how it works?

A. The Big White Wall (www.bigwhitewall.com/landing-pages/landingv3. aspx?ReturnUrl=%2f#.VcjFGhNViko) provides a safe online community of people as a digital support and recovery service for people who are stressed, anxious, feeling low or not coping. At the heart of Big White Wall is its community of members, who support and help each other share what's troubling them in a safe and anonymous environment, with the guidance of trained professionals.

It operates in the same way that a Facebook page offers friends' updates, birthday reminders and contacts to chat with. Big White Wall displays options such as online forums for discussing problems or offering support, tests to understand conditions and even live therapy.

Mindful of service users, the platform offers anonymity, access round the clock and is available via alternative platforms such as tablet and phone via a mobile app. With one in four people suffering with mental health issues such as depression or anxiety, its success rate is impressive: 95% of members reported feeling better after using the service and 80% of users self-managed their issues on the platform.

By the end of its pilot year in 2008, the Big White Wall app had 3000 users and extensive feedback highlighting the value of improving mental well-being.

AppScript is a distribution platform for mobile health technologies, with a system that has scored over 100 000 mobile health apps to enable providers to create their own mHealth apps formulary.

Q2. Can apps be used for diagnostic or assessment purposes?

A. Yes apps can be very useful in these ways. The Mersey Burns tool (www.mersey burns.com/) for example is an app that can be used on an iPhone or tablet to enable clinical staff to quickly and accurately assess burn injuries, and ensure that the correct information follows the patient if they are transferred. It was developed by clinicians.

The app calculates the total body surface area burnt, and amount of fluids the patient requires, as well as incorporating significant factors like a patient's age and height. It can also be used to accurately assess injuries and correctly relay vital information to burns specialists elsewhere, prior to a patient arriving.

References

1. Monitor Deloitte. *Digital Health in the UK: an industry study for the Office of Life Sciences.* London: Deloitte; 2015. Available at: www.deloitte.co.uk/
2. Armstrong S. Which app should I use? *BMJ.* 2015; **351**: h4597. doi: 10.1136bmj.h4597.
3. Medicines and Healthcare Products Regulatory Agency (MHRA). *Medical Device Stand-Alone Software Including Apps.* London: MHRA; 2014. Available at: www.gov.uk/government/publications/medical-devices-software-applications-apps
4. Royal College of Physicians (RCP). *Using Apps in Clinical Practice: important things that you need to know about apps and CE marking.* London: RCP; 2015. Available at: www.rcplondon.ac.uk/file/175/download?token=5nTJceC1
5. Research2guidance. *mHealth App Developer Economics 2014: the state of the art of mHealth app publishing.* Berlin: Research2guidance; 2014. Available at: http://research2guidance.com/r2g/research2guidance-mHealth-App-Developer-Economics-2014.pdf
6. eMarketer. *Worldwide Smartphone Usage to Grow 25% in 2014: nine countries to surpass 50% smartphone penetration this year.* New York, NY: eMarketer. Available at: www.emarketer.com/Article/Worldwide-Smartphone-Usage-Grow-25-2014/1010920
7. Taylor K. *Connected Health: how digital technology is transforming health and social care.* London: Deloitte Centre for Health Solutions; 2015. Available at: www2.deloitte.com/uk/en/pages/life-sciences-and-healthcare/articles/connected-health.html
8. PushDoctor.co.uk. *Last Night the Internet Saved My Life: digital health report 2015.* Manchester: Push Dr; 2015. Available at: https://www.pushdoctor.co.uk/digital-health-report/
9. Lewis T, Wyatt J. mHealth and mobile medical apps: a framework to assess risk and promote safer use. *J Med Internet Res.* 2014; **16**: e210. doi:10.2196/jmir.3133.
10. Husain I, Spence D. Can healthy people benefit from health apps? *BMJ.* 2015; **350**: h1887. doi: 10.1136/bmj.h1887.
11. Local Government Association. *Transforming Local Public Services: using technology and digital tools and approaches.* London: Local Government Association; 2014. Available at: www.local.gov.uk

Chapter 7

Use social media? Get the benefits but minimise risks

Marc Schmid

Will social media not open the floodgates for people to criticise our organisation? How will we moderate negative posts? How will I find the time? These types of questions commonly arise during discussions as to whether an NHS organisation or local authority should embrace social media and regard it as a key channel with which to engage with service users. Sadly, in many instances, this discussion is all that needs to happen to bring a halt to its use before it has even started. Senior managers may offer a multitude of excuses as to why social media shouldn't be used – security risk, reputational risk, too time consuming, the domain of the young etc. But while there is a need to understand the risks, and agree that social media should never replace all other modes of communication, it will be detrimental to any organisation if it simply ignores the advantages of using social media to engage with its population.

An example of this can be seen with YouTube. Many health and social care organisations ban staff from accessing YouTube. However, YouTube can be a powerful tool that disgruntled patients use to get their voice heard as in Example 7.1.

The point illustrated here is that whether an organisation wishes to use social media or not, there is always a chance that it will appear there anyway. The risk is that it may be on a site over which the organisation has no real control or ability to engage patients or service users. A patient can now 'check in' to a social media site when they are waiting for a doctor's appointment and create a profile on the practice's behalf. Having your own well-planned, helpful social media profile can counter this by offering both happy or disgruntled patients and service users not only a helpful medium to speak about their experiences but one which affords the NHS or local authority a right of reply. So listen to patient feedback, monitor online forums and references to your practice or organisation or your name; respond appropriately online, respecting patient confidentiality; and seek to have inappropriate comments removed.

EXAMPLE 7.1   The power of defamation by social media

A patient at Eastbourne District General Hospital was unhappy when he witnessed the same staff cleaning toilets and serving food. He says he complained to the hospital but did not receive an answer. As a recording studio executive, he therefore decided to turn his attention to social media and wrote a song called 'Eastbourne Hospital' which he uploaded to YouTube. This not only built up a following online but was subsequently spotted in mainstream media; see www.bbc.co.uk/news/uk-england-sussex-18366651

More UK adults, especially older adults, are now going online, using a range of devices

According to Ofcom's *Adults' Media Use and Attitudes Report*[1] over eight in ten (83%) adults go online using any type of device in any location. Nearly all 16–24 year olds and 25–34 year olds are now online (98%), and there has been a 9% increase in those aged 65+ years ever going online (42% vs. 33% in 2012).

The number of adults using tablets to go online has almost doubled, from 16% in 2012 to 30% in 2013. While almost all age groups are more likely than previously to use tablets in this way, use by those aged 35–64 years has doubled, while use by 65–74s has trebled, from 5% to 17%.

Six in ten UK adults (62%) now use a smartphone, an increase from 54% in 2012. This increase is driven by 25–34s and 45–54s, and those aged 65–74 are almost twice as likely to use a smartphone now compared to 2012 (20% vs. 12%). The report from the Deloitte Centre for Health Solutions suggests that smartphone penetration is now around 70% of the UK population.[2]

Social media usage

According to Ofcom,[1] two-thirds (66%) of online adults say they have a current social networking site profile, unchanged since 2012 (64%). Nearly all with a current profile (96%) have one on Facebook.[3] Three in ten social networkers say they have a Twitter profile, and one in five says they have YouTube (22%) or WhatsApp (20%) profiles. Social networking overall remains a popular pastime, with 60% of users visiting sites more than once a day, an increase from 50% in 2012, and with 83% of 16–24 year olds doing so (69% in 2012).

Twitter users are the most likely to say they follow friends (72%) and then celebrities (45%) and news (also 45%), followed by hobbies and interests (33%). On average, Twitter users say they follow 146 people or organisations, and have 97 followers. Interestingly, the number of SMSs or MMSs sent on average per month, per user, fell from 227 in 2013 to 170 in 2014, which could signal a gradual shift away from texting towards instant messaging via social media channels.

Over the last decade, there has been a significant global increase in social media usage. In the UK there has been a 47% increase in social media usage since 2007.[4]

Half of the world's estimated online population now checks in to the social networking giant Facebook at least once a month. Facebook revealed in its second-quarter 2015 report that the number of people who use it at least monthly grew 13% to 1.49 billion in the 3 months to the end of June. The number is equal to half of the estimated 3 billion people who use the Internet worldwide. Of those users, it is said that 65% were now accessing Facebook daily.[3]

Social media can contribute to behavioural change by making information more accessible; enabling information to be personalised to more suitable types and formats, and providing consumers with motivational messages or reminders based on their targets or goals. Dr Welton, a GP at Trent Vale Medical Practice in Stoke-on-Trent, recorded short stroke awareness videos which include the signs of stroke, side effects of stroke and lifestyle choices that can lead to stroke. This handy advice is all provided through the practice's public facing Facebook page and has had impressive engagement results.

So who uses social media to obtain health information?

A national survey on the use of social media by people with chronic health conditions[5] describes the substantive extent of peer-to-peer help in place among people living with chronic conditions. One in four Internet users living with high blood pressure, diabetes, heart conditions, lung conditions, cancer or some other chronic ailment (23%) said they have gone online to find others with similar health concerns. By contrast, 15% of Internet users who reported having no chronic conditions had sought such help online. Other groups who were likely to look online for people who share their same health concerns included Internet users who: are caring for a loved one; had had a medical crisis in the past year; had experienced a significant change in their physical health, such as weight loss or gain, pregnancy, or quitting smoking.

This presents a challenge for the NHS. By ignoring such online health discussions the health system runs the risk of allowing well-meaning but unqualified amateurs to offer health advice to others. In one private group created by patients living in Lancashire, members have actually discussed sharing medication when one person's medication has run out. Box 7.1 shows a snapshot of a question asked by a patient in a popular asthma group.

BOX 7.1

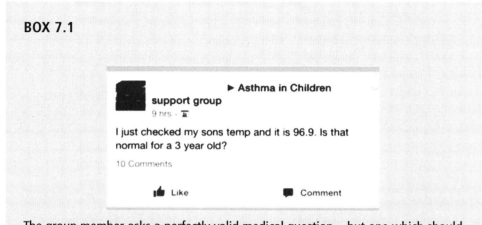

The group member asks a perfectly valid medical question – but one which should be directed at someone with a medical background rather than a Facebook 'friend'. In this instance, the answers were sensible and directed the individual to the NHS Choices website, but there are examples out there of people offering unqualified advice.

Not only might this poor advice or bad practice result in increased demand being placed on an already stretched health or social care system, but it presents a risk of malicious interference or use by people wishing to sell unlicensed medical products such as diet pills or herbal remedies. The flipside of this is that these patient-led community groups offer a powerful peer-to-peer support

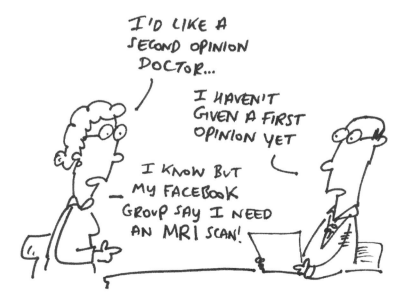

network where patients provide real-life commentary on their experiences for the benefit of others. A great example of this is the 'Living with anxiety' Facebook group where people post personal video clips or 'selfies' explaining the nature of their anxiety as well as how they manage it: www.facebook.com/groups/Depressionanxietymentalhealth/. This group operates in much the same way as a therapy group where people offer their own experiences. These powerful pen pictures of their anxiety provide reassurance to others in the group that they are not alone.

Some of these online Facebook groups have an international following; others might operate within geographical boundaries such as www.facebook.com/groups/lancashire.cumbria.anxiety/?fref=ts. Either way, they can offer a powerful method of supporting people with health concerns in the comfort of their home – as in the case study in Example 7.2. Social media allows communities of people with similar conditions to come together and exchange information or share their experiences. So a health professional's participant role is more that of a guide or interpreter rather than the sole supplier of knowledge about the condition being focused on. At the Royal Stoke University Hospital, clinicians have developed closed Facebook patient groups for a variety of conditions or services. These include multiple sclerosis, atrial fibrillation, stroke, asthma and cardiac rehabilitation.

EXAMPLE 7.2 How a closed Facebook group helped with weight management

The Furlong Medical Centre in Stoke-on-Trent has developed a closed Facebook group linked to its weight management clinic. Patients wishing to receive advice and support from nursing staff can join the closed Facebook group. By creating a closed community of citizens (registered with the practice) who are experiencing the same support, the use of social media has created an environment through which the patients motivate each other. As opposed to a page where posts are filtered resulting in only a proportion of Facebook fans receiving the updates, everyone in the group receives a notification when one of the nurses uploads health information.

Getting started: develop your social media strategy using the five 'Ws'

So if you are considering using social media where do you begin?

Before you use social media in any health setting you need to develop a basic strategy to allow you to focus your social media intervention appropriately and ensure that you allow time to evaluate its effectiveness. To help with this, focus on Table 7.1, which uses a simple 'five Ws' approach that, once completed, you can action to enable you to get the best out of using social media.

TABLE 7.1 The five 'Ws'

Why are you using social media? Are you clear on what outcomes you want to achieve?
What evaluation measures do you have in place to measure your activity? Social media may be free to set up but you should allow for ongoing staff time to manage, moderate and measure the usage
Which groups of people are you targeting?
Where will you find them? There is no point creating a platform where most of its audience is aged over 25 years old if you are looking to engage with 16–24 year olds. Do your research first
Who is going to set up and manage these channels and moderate them? Practices or teams who actively use social media need to ensure that a few staff have the skills to manage the online pages as necessary

In Stoke-on-Trent the majority of GP practices use social media to engage with patients. A local programme included training and support materials for social media being offered to the 52 practices. The most popular form of social media adopted is Facebook but other channels include Twitter and YouTube. The topics discussed on Facebook range from simple health messages to the publication of did not attend (DNA) data and consultations on appointment and telephone systems. Posts are scheduled in advance to be released in the evenings and the moderation of the site is managed through set times across the week. Example 7.3 reports the vast reach to the local population via social media.

EXAMPLE 7.3   Supporting local general practices to use social media

One practice manager, Jane Cope from Goldenhill Medical Centre in North Staffordshire, said, 'We use Facebook as an opportunity to advertise and educate patients on seasonal topics, i.e. influenza vaccines in the winter, holiday vaccinations in the summer etc. and also other information that would be of benefit to patients. It is good to receive feedback from patients. Fortunately all the feedback received so far has been favourable, which is great for staff morale. Should an adverse comment ever be added, we would have the opportunity to take remedial action proactively. As technology develops and more patients use the Web to communicate, we as a forward-thinking practice see Facebook as a new innovative tool with which to communicate and educate our patients.'

Over half of the practices in Stoke-on-Trent now regularly use social media. While there is a common set of rules determining how practices operate across social media, each practice is left to develop its own channels and decide how creative it wants to be. They have all found considerable appetite among patients for engaging with practices and clinics online. In a recent six-month period, of the 30 practices now using social media, the reach was over 200 000 people with more than 12 000 engaged patients regularly interacting with their pages. One practice posted a new YouTube video advertising the range of services it offers and reached 7808 patients in one week thanks to 91 'likes', 57 'comments' and 32 'shares' (Facebook Insights).

In terms of the demographics of patients, 85% of the patient population engaging with the practices via social media are female. Interestingly, 66% of patient users are between 25 and 55 years old and there are more users over 55 years engaging with practices on social media than there are under 25 years old. You need to ask yourself why this should surprise us. Older people are increasingly embracing technology such as tablets and smartphones and as such will migrate onto sites such as Facebook so they can keep in touch with family. In Lancashire, 75-year-old Frances Buckle moved from the town she had grown up in (Blackburn) to a neighbouring town that she had no real experience of (Leyland). She was bought an iPad and explains how she moved on to Facebook:

> I first used the iPad to read the Lancashire Telegraph as I thought it offered the best way of me staying in touch with news in Blackburn. However, I set up a Facebook account so I could keep in touch with my children and grandchildren and began "liking" groups such as photos of Blackburn of old. I have had chats with people I have not spoken to in years in these groups and love using Facebook to keep in touch with friends, family and news from where I've spent most of my life. Without Facebook, I would have certainly felt more isolated in a new town.

Be creative

Using social media to engage with patients is simple once you have established who your audience is and what you want to achieve. What social media won't do is to share your content with thousands of people without you having given some thought to what messages you are communicating. The most effective way of doing this is for you to put yourself in the shoes of the person using your site and imagine what they would be likely to read and share.

Example 7.4 demonstrates how you can bring patients on board as your allies through social media.

EXAMPLE 7.4   Extending patient participation in service planning

Belgrave Medical Centre had a small patient participation group (PPG) that didn't fully represent the demographics of its patient community. It generally contained older patients who were retired and therefore able to dedicate more of their time than younger, employed people. The practice had a large number of younger mothers whom it wanted to encourage to become members of the PPG but due to childcare issues could not persuade them to join. A closed PPG Facebook group was created with invitations sent out via Facebook to join. The group which has over 40 members runs in parallel to the original PPG thus giving the practice a wider range of views. An interview with the practice manager, Jenny Woodfint, as to how they manage the Facebook PPG can be found on www.digitalhealthsot.nhs.uk

Jenny describes her experience of Facebook as: 'a most useful tool to the practice, enabling us to give information to patients in a timely manner, promote general health information and improve patient participation. In order to get started, the practice set up an administrator account and then created a page accessible by all and also a closed group to allow us to develop our PPG to encourage groups of patients whom we had difficulty engaging with to participate. Once set up we then promoted the page through posters and information on prescriptions and it quickly took off with the number of likes increasing on a daily basis.

'With regard to our page there is some day-to-day management of the site required but this is just a few minutes each day; this involves someone viewing Facebook daily for comments and responding to the comments. On a monthly basis the practice agrees the priorities for information to be transferred and this is usually based on seasonal topics such as sunburn or barbecue safety in summer and flu vaccination or childhood illnesses in the winter. These are then set up as scheduled posts which automatically post to our site on the dates we agree. We take care to post at key times such as evenings and weekends so that the information is seen by a large number of people.

'With regard to our PPG closed group, this runs in parallel with our face-to-face meeting group and the same information is shared with both groups and comments invited. This has allowed us to expand the demographics of our PPG considerably, attracting youngsters and parents who weren't able to attend our face-to-face meetings. We have found that through social media people will make comments both good and bad. Below are examples of the two extremes that we have been sent:

- "Couldn't agree more with XXXXX about this practice being one of the best. I hear my colleagues complaining all the time about how they wait a week for appointments or can't get through to their surgery on the telephone."
- "This is the most disgusting practice and the practice manager is a waste of space."

'We have a policy to respond to all comments, thanking people for the positive comments they make and for any suggestions and also apologising to those complaining that we have not met the standards they expect and explaining what they should do next to take the matter further. A standardised approach is needed to this to avoid any potential problems and potential breaches of confidentiality as people expand on their comments.

'Facebook has worked really well for the practice; it has been an asset for the transfer of information and expanding our PPG. Initially we were concerned about the negative comments but these should be embraced and used as learning opportunities. Facebook has been a real asset to our service.'

Organisations frequently make the mistake of assuming that all content is treated the same and therefore that just by posting something you can circulate

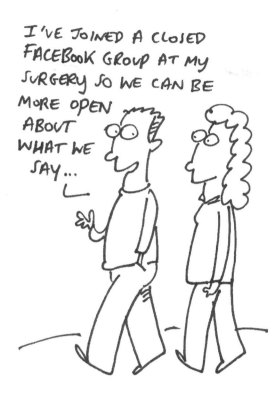

this to thousands of eager social media users. This is simply not the case. Only content considered to be of interest to the user will make an impact. For example, posting a link to the minutes of last month's PPG meeting will have no impact whatsoever. However, explaining how many appointments have been lost by people failing to turn up and the impact that this is having on services will spark an online discussion and in turn ensure that your reach via social media is bigger. Similarly, structuring your social media activity around events and topical issues will help. If there is a lot of national media focus on flu then updates on flu vaccines, clinics or general health tips will have more of an impact. Some of the best practices have created calendars of issues and will schedule their posts in advance. This could include health and diet tips in January when people are making New Year resolutions to lose weight or stop smoking.

The key to success is creativity. Social media will bring a personality to an organisation and some familiarity which will help to soften any negative attitudes that may exist. People are less likely to be hostile to an organisation if they feel as though they are addressing a person. This is why organisations like Tesco and Virgin Trains spend a lot of time developing their social media profiles as part of their customer services.

Creating advocates

The real success of using social media in health or social care can be seen by the creation of advocates. One of the most powerful impacts of social media in any organisation is when users begin to respond on its behalf. These 'external' posts are far more powerful than anything the organisation itself can do and will only come about once a proper relationship between an organisation and its social media followers has developed. This is why a great deal of time and effort needs to be spent on generating conversations and most importantly responding to social media posts. Blackburn with Darwen Council created a winter Facebook page several years ago called BwD Winter. These pages were used to provide useful advice on winter weather disruption but invariably attracted a lot of criticism from residents who used it to vent frustration on a perceived lack of gritting. The council persevered, however, and the site has become a fantastic 'go to' site for weather impact updates all year round. In the winter, the posts are managed by the highways teams who will post gritting route updates in real time as well as live weather updates. By doing this, every critical comment now generates multiple supportive comments from people with no links to the council. On 26 December 2015 during the flood problems, a single post reporting road closures generated over 200 shares, over 23 000 post clicks and a reach of over 120 000 people.

There are some excellent examples where patients defend a GP practice when complaints are posted about the availability of appointments as well as adding glowing praise for practice staff in response to posts about customer services. An important point to remember is that a disgruntled patient will be posting negative comments anyway regardless of whether the organisation is using social media or not. By engaging with social media an organisation can try to manage the complaint and take it offline. This approach is adopted by companies such as Nissan which invest a great deal of time and energy into turning owners into advocates by creating brand loyalty. They strive to create what they call brand evangelists – people who will share the brand's story with others and defend the brand. This can also be achieved by health organisations such as GP practices and hospitals. By capturing positive experiences through social media and nurturing relationships, advocates can be developed. It is important to note, however, that if there is a barrage of complaints you must check whether there are underlying problems causing it and resolve them.

Dealing with difficult posts

If any health or social care organisation expects to maximise the benefit of social media it needs to avoid the temptation to simply delete any comments that it rates as negative or worse and get drawn into a public tit for tat. It needs to adopt a grown-up approach and understand that someone posting a negative remark should not automatically mean that the comment should be removed. Constructive criticism is no bad thing and any response acknowledging a complaint and pledging to look into it can be a powerful plus in terms of developing advocates and supporters. The simplest way of managing negative posts is to contact the complainant directly by messaging them and inviting them to make the complaint in person. By doing this you are asking them to consider whether they are serious or not, as well as reassuring them that you are taking their complaint seriously and are prepared to listen. It can often be the case that critics can be turned into advocates simply by you responding to a complaint effectively.

Conflict between professional and personal

While your working hours might generally end at 5–6 p.m., social media changes the rules a little. If you can easily be identified as working for the NHS or social care, your behaviour there will reflect on the NHS or local authority in general, whether you want it to or not. You have no control over people's perceptions of you and, additionally, you have a responsibility to ensure that problems and issues at work do not leak over into your use of social media. In addition, it can actually be beneficial to your professional use of social media to introduce some of your personal interests in order to prevent yourself looking robotic. Here are some basic tips on preventing mishaps:

Do	Don't
Put a disclaimer on any account where you speak about your job role or the NHS stating that the opinions are your own and not those of your employer. This includes Facebook if you identify on there that you work for the NHS	Assume hiding a comment behind a privacy setting means it will never see the light of day. It's easy for people to take a screenshot with your words in black and white
Understand that this disclaimer will not protect you from your public comments being taken out of context as the Press Complaints Commission recently ruled	Tag inappropriate photos on Facebook which are public (and if they're not, beware of the 'friends of friends' sharing setting)
Understand that as soon as you make a post in your work capacity on your personal account, you have crossed the line in relation to the professional guidelines – see FAQ 1	Disclose any confidential data or patient information online
Think about your posts from a patient or service user perspective. Is this something they would be interested in reading and sharing with their friends?	Make disparaging remarks about people you work with or the public you come into contact with at work, even if your privacy settings are closed
Ensure that staff using social media have had some training and are comfortable using social media	Post anything privately you would not be happy showing to your line manager or saying to your line manager's or colleague's face

Maintaining a healthy personal online profile

Whether you work in health or social care or not, your personal online profile can have a significant effect on how others perceive you regardless of how well up to speed you are with your settings. There are some simple rules that you should follow, though, to help you to maintain a healthy online profile.

1. Treat people with respect

On the Internet, people hide behind a veil of anonymity to attack, slander and discredit people whom they don't like. With social media networks and blogs, it's easy to find a stranger to pick on. The number one rule therefore is to treat people with respect. There is a great online video called *Digital Dirt Sticks* at www.youtube.com/watch?v=JJfw3xt4emY in which a job applicant is humiliated by a potential employer after she rooted out comments the girl had made on Facebook about another girl. Not surprisingly she doesn't get the job!

2. Don't spread gossip

Thanks to websites like Twitter, breaking news can reach millions of people within seconds. In some cases, this is a good thing. Social media users are among the first to learn about important events and news. When the news is false, however, the speed of social media can get people into all sorts of bother.

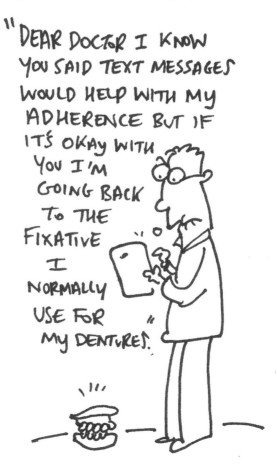

A good rule is to be sceptical of what you read online. Check your facts before you share that information. If the information is found to be libellous, it will not be a defence to claim that you did not understand what you were doing. Ask yourself this – would my employer be happy if I shared this information?

3. Keep private information private

Some companies focus their entire business model on searching social networking websites for personal information and then compiling it to sell to marketeers. That's why private information online should stay private. Another good tip is to avoid the photos on Facebook that encourage large numbers of people to share them – these are often scams with the intention of selling the information on. Most importantly, never share any health data or information from within your own organisation – confidential information should remain just that.

4. Google yourself

Employers will often do it, so why don't you? Having a look at your online profile will help you to understand what you look like to others. Then if you want to, you can plan to modify your profile or extend it.

5. Think about the future

Things that you share online are like digital tattoos; they're there forever. Look at yourself from the outside and remove anything from your own social media sites that you think might paint you in an awkward light in the future. Imagine the embarrassment of a smoking cessation health worker having photos on their Facebook pages of them smoking – no matter how old they are. There may be perfectly rational explanations, but unfortunately in the online world the messages portrayed are often seen as black or white.

Growing 'participatients'

Julia Manning highlighted the advantages of technology enabled care in empowering patients in learning about their conditions so that they can take real shared responsibility for their own management – in her foreword inventing the term 'participatients'. A research focus on the experiences of young people with diabetes has illustrated how they as patients 'actively and effortlessly negotiated between evidence-informed, professionally produced content and user-generated content'. They navigated between various sources of clinical and condition-specific information including professionally produced websites and user-generated content. Many used these and social media 'to inform self-management strategies, drawing on others' experiences or niche content brought together by issue-specific online communities'.[6]

FAQs

Q1. I'm a nurse. Is there any special guidance on social media for me in my professional role?

A. Yes, the Nursing and Midwifery Council has published useful guidance.[7] Another useful guidance document is the *Social Media Highway Code* published by the Royal College of General Practitioners.[8]

Q2. How can I learn what is good practice so that I can start using Twitter?

A. There are some great examples out there of organisations using Twitter effectively as part of their customer services. As previously mentioned, Tesco is very good at responding to queries on Twitter but a quick search of any household name companies will usually find they are using it as a valuable tool to improve customer services. A good test is to look at their tweets and see if they are automated responses or genuinely providing support to the customer. NHS Choices has a great Twitter feed which provides daily health advice on a range of topics. These tweets provide useful content and links which can be posted on other sites such as Facebook.

Q3. Where can I find help and advice which can support our use of social media?

A. The website www.digitalhealthsot.nhs.uk has some valuable support documents to help you use social media safely. There is a digital toolkit as well as staff guides and user guides which can all be downloaded. There is also a useful Twitter account called @digihealth_ that will provide help and support for organisations wishing to use social media.

References

1. Ofcom. *Adults' Media Use and Attitudes Report*. London: Ofcom; 2014. Available at: http://stakeholders.ofcom.org.uk/binaries/research/media-literacy/adults-2014/2014_Adults_report.pdf
2. Taylor K. *Connected Health: how digital technology is transforming health and social care*. London: Deloitte Centre for Health Solutions; 2015. Available at: www.deloitte.co.uk/centreforhealthsolutions
3. Facebook. *Facebook Reports Second Quarter 2015 Results*. Menlo Park, CA: Facebook; 2015. Available at: http://investor.fb.com/releasedetail.cfm?ReleaseID=924562
4. Dutton WH, Blank G. *Next Generation Users: the Internet in Britain*. Oxford: Oxford Internet Institute; 2011. Available at: www.oii.ox.ac.uk/publications/oxis2011_report.pdf
5. Fox S. *Peer to Peer Healthcare*. Washington DC: Pew Internet and American Life Project; 2011. Available at: www.pewInternet.org/2011/02/28/peer-to-peer-health-care-2/
6. Fergie G, Hilton S, Hunt K. Young adults' experiences of seeking online information about diabetes and mental health in the age of social media. *Health Expect*. 2015 8 December. doi: 10.1111/hex.12430.

7. Nursing and Midwifery Council (NMC). *Guidance on Using Social Media Responsibly*. London: NMC; 2015. Available at: www.nmc.org.uk/standards/guidance/social-networking-guidance/
8. Royal College of General Practitioners (RCGP). *Social Media Highway Code*. London: RCGP; 2013. Available at: www.rcgp.org.uk

Part Two

Making digital healthcare happen

Chapter 8

Patient and public perspectives: listen and communicate well

Jayne Birch-Jones, Dr Ruth Chambers

Do people want technology enabled care services (TECS)?

Well, it's usual now for people to interact with digital services for banking, shopping or booking holidays – so why is it not the norm for them to interact with NHS and social care services in similar online ways? Many health and social care professionals and staff are frustrated by the lack of technology infrastructure and support for interoperability between teams in different care settings, and between health and care professionals with patients or service users.

Patient representatives do support the potential benefits for digital care – but warn them that it may be difficult for some vulnerable people with, for example, dementia or learning disabilities, to learn to adapt to using the Internet and other digital modes of delivery of care. There are lots of examples, though, where TECS have helped these population groups, so one of the current challenges is to give NHS and social care leaders confidence that online services have a major part to play in health and social care service provision. More than 80% of households in England are thought to have Internet access, so there are lots of opportunities to develop online access to care.[1]

Listening to patients' experience

So what difference does patient and public involvement in the implementation of TECS make? How can you organise it and what are the benefits? A patient champion shares his experience in the case study in Example 8.1. His story is inspirational. It demonstrates the power of patient stories as an effective communication conduit; you could mirror this when you're implementing TECS in your own health or social care setting.

EXAMPLE 8.1   'Flo telehealth saved my life' by Josh Youd, Flo champion and advocate

'Being a type one diabetic is tough, but is it not amazing when something simple and extraordinary suddenly pops along to save the day? Well, this is what happened to me roughly three years ago. Its name is Flo (that is a simple telehealth programme via SMS texting that can work on any type of mobile phone) and I can definitely say Flo has saved my life!

'I was in a very bad place and I wasn't looking after myself. My mum was at her wits' end and my nurse was running out of ideas to motivate me. She asked me if I would talk to a lady from a telehealth project, Jayne. I did and after a bit of discussion I thought, well, what have I got to lose – I'll have a go. After being enrolled onto the Flo system, changes began immediately. Flo's constant messages turned on my engines and made me suddenly aware that I had to be responsive to the rapid rises in my blood sugar levels. After a short period of time I noticed positive changes in my moods and how I felt about life in general. After a few months of using Flo, I really felt the benefit of my diabetes being better controlled through the daily monitoring and support messages via Flo. I was approached by the local Flo team to be a patient champion. I was asked to tell my story, participating in both staff and public events and meetings when I was free (and feeling well enough).

'I quickly agreed as I felt it was important to give something back to the NHS as it has been my cornerstone through seven years of diabetes. Wanting to have some kind of identification, the team provided me with a "Flo super user" baseball cap for me to wear when working with them!

'I started participating in a few local meetings and group talks with other NHS staff. My self-assurance grew, particularly after I encountered a GP who was very negative about Flo. We had a very constructive conversation about the use of Flo from the perspective of a patient. I am proud to say that the upshot was that he went away thinking very differently. I was slightly worried that I may have overstepped the mark, but when I turned round to talk to the team, they were wide eyed in admiration at how I had handled the situation.

'Having proven my ability to stand my ground (professionally and politely of course!), I was invited to take part in a webinar run by the Health and Social Care Information Centre in Leeds, about increasing patient self-management and compliance. Although I was very nervous, taking part gave me great confidence after receiving really good feedback and lots of questions.

'Not long after, I took part in my first major face-to-face event at the DW Stadium, home of Wigan Athletic Football Club and Wigan Warriors. The day started off rather shakily for me as I was not feeling well. But once I took to the stage to tell my Flo story to a large audience of senior managers, GPs and other staff, I was soon positively distracted! I have to admit I got teary eyed, on receiving a rapturous standing applause. From there on, it started a busy road to my participation at more national events.

'Another very memorable event was meeting some delegates on an exchange visit with the Department of Veterans Affairs (VA) from the USA. The doctors were very interested in both how Flo was helping me to manage my diabetes better and also the role I played with the team. I treasure the VA's hat that they sent me on their return home!

'The team and I got lots of interest and enquiries about my role, including from the East Midlands Academic Health Science Network. They were really keen to spread my story and experience and asked if I would make a short film that could be used across the NHS and this was included on their website. I have since made several films including one for the Digital Health NHS Stoke-on-Trent website[2] and another for the Mid Nottinghamshire Better Together Programme (for whom I'm also a patient champion). To me, the most important and challenging film I've made was a 60-second clip which was included in the team's presentation that they had to provide when they were shortlisted in the telehealth category of the HSJ Value in Healthcare award.

'I was approached through the Mansfield and Ashfield CCG's communication team by a journalist from the local newspaper *The Chad* and asked to tell my Flo story. This was a great experience and I was really pleased with the finished article. It made a great change to read a positive news item in my local paper!

'As if all this activity was not exciting enough, imagine how I felt when I was invited with Jayne, the programme manager, and a nurse to visit Downing Street to talk about Flo. Yes, you read it right – the big place itself. I was nervous; I am not going to lie. It's not every day I am invited to meet the Minister for Policy. The day went very well and he was impressed with how simple and effective the system was. And so our team went home in extremely high spirits. It was a privilege and honour to support the Flo team.

'Last autumn, while supporting the team at one of the CCG's Annual General Meetings, I was gobsmacked to say the least to be presented with a Mansfield and Ashfield CCG Excellence in Engagement Award. This was in recognition of my contribution to the team over the last year. I was absolutely thrilled and humbled. It feels like there is always something exciting round the corner, which is really important for me as my general health, despite Flo's help, is not always great.

'Recently I have been to some other great events; for example, I was invited to the King Power Stadium in Leicester to present on my Flo experience in relation to medication compliance. This was another great privilege as I love telling people how amazing this system is and how it has pretty much saved my life.

'Imagine my delight when Jayne turned up with a book[3] for me a month or so back, by the infamous Dr Phil Hammond, that included my case study "It's a lot easier having a nurse in your pocket!" I was ecstatic as anyone else would be.

'Just to put all this in perspective, in the year before I started using Flo I had

46 admissions to hospital in 2011; that reduced to just a handful the year after. Now and in the future, things are looking up, as my Lady Flo is always in my pocket and by my side.

'On a very last note (I promise) I just want to say … Simplicity is Best.'

Promoting patient empowerment and self-care

Josh relays a very powerful case study of what can be achieved by patient empowerment – improving his self-care and involving Josh in service redesign and development on an organisational scale. The aims of promoting self-care among your patients or the local population are to encourage individual people to:

> **P**: **P**revent the condition developing
> **A**: **A**wait resolution of the symptoms
> **R**: use self-care skills for **R**elief of symptoms
> **T**: learn to **T**olerate symptoms that do not resolve or cannot be reasonably alleviated.[4]

The size of each quadrant in Figure 8.1 will depend on the specific level and range of self-care skills for a particular condition.

P Prevent the condition developing	**A** Await resolution of the symptoms
R Use self-care skills for Relief of symptoms	**T** Learn to Tolerate symptoms that do not resolve or cannot be reasonably alleviated

FIGURE 8.1 Pathways for self-care

Enhance the level of self-care skills of individuals and self-care support that you provide by considering each component. Push the boundaries of self-care to the maximum that is safe for your individual patients and affordable in terms of resources such as time and capacity of you and your team. Some self-care support approaches will focus on one of the quadrants. Others may have more than one component in the total intervention.

Self-management

Self-management support and patient education are core to enabling individual patients to share management of best practice in care of their long-term conditions or take responsibility to combat unhealthy lifestyle habits. Engaging people in interventions to support their self-management often fails to show significant improvements in care if their clinicians are not motivated to educate and upskill individual patients. So we need service delivery models which are easy for health and social care teams to adopt and that require minimal change in their everyday workload and, ideally, an overall reduction. Mobile technology is now a well-proven conduit to drive positive self-management behaviours in such ways as can be integrated into patients' lives – as with Josh in the case study.

So you'll encourage behaviour change via self-management by shared care between patient or service user and health or care professional by:

- establishing a shared agenda – what it is that you are both focusing on
- setting goals – agreed by patient and carer as being achievable and beneficial
- following up how well those goals are achieved, or agree other linked goals if progress is slow or the self-management doesn't work out as planned or – better still – goals are attained so fast that you can agree another set.

Engaging individual patients in use of TECS

To maximise engagement and satisfaction of both patients and professionals the type of TECS selected should be for the right patients by the right professionals using the service in the right circumstances to address a problem identified by clinicians and patient users. Remember that 'one size does not fit all' and you should be selective when offering patients a particular mode of delivery of care to ensure that they are receptive to, and have confidence in, remote management of their condition rather than traditional face-to-face care methods.

Sharing decision making

As a health or social care professional you should respect the values and beliefs of patients and not try to impose your own attitudes upon them. A potential imbalance of power is created by your superior knowledge as the provider of services. Shared decision making is the middle ground between informed choice, where decisions are left entirely to the patient, and traditional, paternalistic medical decision making. It involves two-way information giving (clinical and personal) between the clinician and patient concerning all options available, with the final decision being made jointly with both parties in total agreement.

To share information and relate well requires you to consider how you interact with a patient in respect of:

- *partnership*: help for someone with a problem through partnership between that person and professionals
- *empowerment*: help for those with problems to find the best ways of helping themselves
- *judgement*: beware of judgement – the person with the problem is the only one who really understands their experience and problem
- *values*: people's values and priorities change with time; they may be quite different from your values, but no less valid
- *autonomy*: autonomy should be a fundamental right of everyone. Illness, disability, low income, unemployment and other forms of social exclusion mean a loss of some aspects of autonomy in society
- *listening*: active non-judgemental listening is core to helping people, and crucial to gain an understanding of people with problems
- *shared decision making*: people with ongoing problems need to be able to take their own decisions about the care of their clinical condition, based on expert information communicated to them by professionals.

An engaged patient is more likely to adhere to medication or other treatment interventions – because of the rapport created with their care professional and their improved understanding of their condition or likely outcomes of their behaviour. So the health or social care professional needs to establish:

- a shared approach to planning and managing the condition or behaviour
- shared goal setting
- follow-up of progress in relation to agreed goals and ongoing care.

The shared goals and plans need to be person centred – and coordinated across different providers of care and take into account co-morbidities or various adverse lifestyle habits that the person is hoping to redress. In general feedback from patients or service users is that they welcome individualised goals that are set to support them to improve their health, and it helps them to feel more in control. This is more about 'concordance' than 'compliance' in that the person understands why the goals need to be set to improve their health and the what and how of doing so, rather than being instructed to simply adhere to clinician-set goals and actions.

The more up-to-date information that a patient receives about their condition, such as bodily measurements (e.g. blood pressure) and test results (e.g. HbA1c and cholesterol for those with diabetes), in the context of the goals agreed in the shared care plan, then the more motivated the patient is likely to be to strive to attain the agreed health-related goals.

User involvement

User involvement and engagement is a key central element for NHS reforms, including the development and adoption of TECS. Solving the issues of public accountability, transparency and equal access all depend on a degree of user involvement.

Services will be better configured around patient and public needs, designed with and for patients and the wider public, to improve people's ability to find their way around the system so they are more likely to be able to access TECS to help them manage their own conditions and improve their overall satisfaction with their health or social care services.

Individual users or members of relevant local voluntary groups or disease-specific groups are ideal for advising on the design and evolution of a local TECS. Hopefully non-executive directors on trust and CCG boards can advise provider and commissioning managers on service redesign, as the TECS are conceived, ordered, launched and deployed.

Social innovation is the key to catalysing how people are involved in their own care and that of others, so improving the quality of their care. Social innovation involves harnessing the power of people – patients, carers, communities and citizens – to improve health.[5]

Communicating with the general public

- **Information:** think what's the best mode of communication or range of types about TECS – for different people with various preferences? Is it a whiteboard animation on a website that takes people through a specific disease-orientated pathway? Is it a simple patient leaflet – with or without cartoons or diagrams that capture the reader's interest or help explain the meaning? Is it a comprehensive website with varied sections that help the online visitor probe more deeply into the content? Is it other sorts of social media such as Facebook (open to all, or closed Facebook group) to which you add regular content and provide oversight and administration? Or would a podcast or YouTube video be better so that viewers can watch and learn, rather than try to read and then drop off to sleep? Or if your information is to be conveyed to the general population at large through the local newspaper, you'll need to find out what the editor wants and conform to their requirements (word length, pitch, scope, focus etc.) to get it accepted for publication.
- **Health literacy:** in essence keep the content as simple and straightforward as possible. Remember that many of those accessing health

and social care with complex health problems or long-term conditions have poor literacy skills. Many will have associated mental health problems (e.g. depression, dementia) that impair their concentration, so they'd be unlikely to plough through a learned essay, and will prefer short sentences with unambiguous content, simple health messages and words of two syllables or fewer where that's possible. Go for the type of language and style likely to suit the typical reader – not too flowery if you're trying to convey health messages. Take care not to use wording that may be misinterpreted, such as 'chronic' which may be understood by lay readers to mean 'serious' rather than 'long lasting' when used to describe a health condition.

- **Get the right sort of help:** if you're inexperienced in writing for the public you could maybe recruit a lay proof reader or expert patient before you finalise the copy – and get their perspectives on content and layout. If you are setting up a website for the general public to use, get a website expert to advise on the layout to create the right sort of eye pattern, to cater for people who are visually impaired with a minimum font size and smart colouring, with short and succinct sections of text that is easily searchable with key terms. It's thought that more than four-fifths of UK households have access to the Internet, so exploit that by making your website more appealing and useful.

- **Grab people's attention:** add debate, analysis and frequently asked questions. Tell the story of the content with an apt headline or title or subheading. Hook the reader with the first sentence – which could be a rhetorical question (Couldn't it?). Add quotations – especially if this is praise of some sort from well-known or trusted people.

- **Writing a patient leaflet:** imagine who the content is for. Use an 'active' voice rather than 'passive' style. Write it or commission it, so that it is angled at the likely recipients and is pitched at the level and range of background knowledge they're likely to have. The ending should capture the solution to the hook question that was posed at the beginning of the article or posted content. Take time to polish the final version – don't rush your first attempt out.

- **Evidence based?** Try to provide trustworthy text in any information you provide or share with individuals. It's your credibility at stake if you're advising that someone reads up on a method of TECS that you're recommending. If you have any conflicts of interest you should declare them in any literature that you write or provide (e.g. if you gain in some way by increasing sales or usage). It may be that you have to include case studies and anecdotes rather than well-grounded research evidence (which does not exist for most modes of TECS – especially as there'll be ongoing technological developments and any published research study is likely to reference old versions of a particular mode of technology). Include relevant and important clinical messages which can be justified by published evidence – so your evidence base of well-grounded research supports best practice in clinical management, rather than use of a particular type of technology. So be clear about any evidence and summarise it succinctly; give sufficient detail but don't drown the reader with lots of data.

- **Interactive?** Invite feedback and get an engaging debate going online. Or write a series of blogs or tweets that relay new research or thinking or signpost people to your information resources or website. You could offer a service such as a learning resource that generates answers to questions or submissions or provides the avenue that takes the user to a type of technology providing interactive care.
- **Understand the effect of your personality on your communication skills:** be aware of the influence of your 'thinking and judging' personality or 'sensing and feeling' traits on how your way of communicating might be perceived by others. If you automatically label someone who is obese as a failure who only has themselves to blame for their associated health conditions, you are likely to disengage them before you've started to inform them about their condition and how TECS might help them to try to change their lifestyle habits or self-manage their condition better. So try to adopt a communication style that is non-judgemental and seek to inform and motivate people to adopt healthy behaviour via their preferred mode of TECS. You can still show your passion for supporting people to regain health and well-being, but in a supportive way rather than a bossy manner. Feel free to give your views but do not come over as an opinionated individual who barks out instructions and doesn't listen.
- **Disclaimer?** If you're giving health messages which might be interpreted as conveying medical advice, you should add a disclaimer. This might simply remind the reader that the information provided is generic and does not replace that which their own doctor or nurse might give them; and that new evidence of best practice is frequently being published and might replace some of the content in your information resource.

FAQs

Q1. Have you advice about the content of a press release?

A. If you're at the stage in your TECS programme of work where you have something new to say, consider triggering a press release about your recent achievement or new offer of care. If you're employed or are contracted to an organisation, seek its help in finalising the press release. Keep it corporate; its media team is probably more savvy than you are in drafting the wording of the press release and getting it out there.

Q2. Have you any concerns about the suitability of TECS for some patients or service users?

A. Some patients may become too obsessed with technology, such as taking their blood pressure night and day to text in when there is no need for that frequency. Clinicians and social workers or family carers should be aware of this kind of reaction in some patients and aid their sensible use of TECS. The type of TECS needs to be selected for the patient's health and care needs, preferences and ability (e.g. cognitive function) and confidence (e.g. operating a tablet, texting responses).

References

1. Ofcom. *Internet Use and Attitudes: 2015 metrics bulletin*. London: Ofcom; 2015. Available at: http://stakeholders.ofcom.org.uk/binaries/research/cmr/cmr15/Internet_use_and_attitudes_bulletin.pdf

2. www.digitalhealthsot.nhs.uk/index.php/clinicians-learning-centre/resources/videos

3. Hammond P. *Staying Alive: how to get the best out of the NHS*. London: Quercus Publishing Ltd; 2015.

4. Chambers R, Wakley G, Blenkinsopp A. *Supporting Self Care in Primary Care*. Abingdon: Radcliffe Publishing; 2006.

5. Bland J, Khan H, Loder J *et al. The NHS in 2030: a vision of a people-powered, knowledge-powered health system*. London: Nesta; 2015. Available at: www.nesta.org.uk/sites/default/files/the-nhs-in-2030.pdf

Chapter 9

Making digital delivery happen in health and social care: at an organisational level

Dr Ruth Chambers

Technology enabled care has become more embedded in all health and social care settings over the last 10 years via self-monitoring or interactive exchange between person and clinician, or using diagnostic or reporting equipment based at the person's home with oversight from their health or social care professional. The widespread rollout of such technology focused on individuals' self-care, prevention of deterioration of long-term conditions and healthy lifestyle habits offers many potential benefits. These include reduction in avoidable hospital (re)admissions, improved quality of life, enhanced patient understanding and self-management of their long-term conditions underpinned by shared care management plans agreed with their clinician, lower mortality rates and reduced costs of acute care. Technology enabled care services (TECS) offer service commissioners and NHS or social care providers the opportunity to transform services and improve the quality and convenience of patient care while at the same time minimising costs of providing care. So we all need to 'create the right

NHS England has requested that Clinical Commissioning Groups (CCGs) complete a 'local digital roadmap' of organisations[2,3] and collaborate in their plan to become 'paper free at the point of care' with fully interoperable digital records and digital transfer of patient information across care settings within their health and care economies. See www.england.nhs.uk/digitaltechnology/info-revolution/digital-roadmaps/

commissioning environment that supports and encourages the innovative use of technology to improve health outcomes, enhances productivity of the NHS/social care workforce and delivers more cost effective services'.[1]

Current challenges

So how do we afford the evolving costs of health and social care for the increasing numbers of elderly people who are living longer with chronic conditions? How do we encourage people to take more responsibility for their health and reasonable control of their own care? How do we empower clinicians to work with other health and social care professionals with the data and information they need about their individual patients at the right time and right setting? What are the productivity opportunities via new models of care, using digital delivery? All of these current society challenges require us to develop deliverable proposals for digital delivery in health and social care that are ambitious but achievable.

How do we change organisational culture so that staff think digital first?

The challenge is to change the general public's attitudes and the culture across the NHS or social care to embed technology in digital delivery and create service transformation of provision of care; this particularly includes public health and lifestyle behaviour. We must take advantage of current opportunities for digital delivery. We need to overcome obstacles such as data sharing about individual patients or service users across care providers, and the absence of Wi-Fi in many health and social care settings.

Empowered patients with access to their health information should be given an opportunity to use this resource to better manage their health. But it will be counterproductive if greater access to information leads to more demands being placed on an already stretched healthcare delivery system.

Create an agreed strategy

Your digital delivery strategy should be focused on your overall goal with a plan to achieve that goal. The key components of developing a strategy include:

- developing your vision and goals
- understanding the current environment in the NHS and social care
- future planning and anticipating the challenges and expectations
- managing change
- leadership
- a road map of your IT infrastructure.[3]

EXAMPLE 9.1   Evolving the strategy of the Staffordshire Digital Health Board

The board was launched in April 2014 and was formed by NHS and local authority leaders from across Staffordshire in recognition of the multi-agency collaboration required to support changes necessary to facilitate delivery of care using modes of digital health. The board has representation from all six CCGs, both unitary local authorities, housing providers, Age UK as a key voluntary sector organisation, the community trust provider (health and social care), both mental health trusts, three acute trust providers, the Commissioning Support Unit and the West Midlands Academic Health Science Network. In late 2014 the board (renamed Technology Enabled Care Services [TECS] Board), with involvement of advisory groups (including patient advisory group), developed its overall strategy focused around the board's agreed main purpose of creating an overall delivery plan through which organisations can begin to implement new technologies and solutions to support the 1.1 million population of Staffordshire and staff who deliver services. In particular the strategy agreed by all member organisations in autumn 2014 focused on extending the use of TECS with a range of digital modalities, supporting more productive working and local service transformation from across the local health economy.

Since then, there has been increasing interest in cross-setting working to promote digital delivery of care – though the impact of the envisaged service transformation has been slower than optimistically set out.

Developing a vision

Your vision needs to be embedded in reality. It should be a clear, shared vision of the future of digital delivery of care that shapes change. So consider the following.

- What are the major trends in society and how will these affect the way you deliver care?
- What will your patients or service users require of us in five years' time?
- What will happen if you stay as you are?
- What critical events that are likely to occur in the future will affect us (e.g. increasing numbers of frail elderly people)?
- How can you capitalise on the increasing capacity and capability of the general public to communicate via digital means?

Your vision underpins the core purpose of your development and implementation of your TECS strategy.

Understanding the environment

A key element in developing your strategy is to map out the current environment in health and social care. All the influences on your organisation (e.g. your local health economy, your practice, your care team) and staff should be considered:

- government bodies
- pressure groups
- media
- patients or service users
- suppliers
- research or evidence of worth of various modes of technology
- laws and regulations, e.g. the Care Act 2014
- policies
- information etc.

You need to understand the key influences on your development of TECS and how they will affect the expectations and requirements for delivery of care by your organisation or team now and in the future (planning for the next five years at least).

Management of the strategy

The logical steps to creating your TECS strategy and managing change are to:

1. engage with stakeholders
2. develop an agreed strategy
3. produce a plan that fits with local or national priorities
4. identify and plan to mitigate risks and issues
5. seek approval from all who will be commissioning or providing the ensuing services
6. implement the strategy or plan in realistic ways with sufficient resources (including funds, training, protected time for staff, integration into service, redesigned delivery pathways).

Change programmes are complex and you should anticipate what actions to include in your implementation plan to increase the likelihood that your TECS strategy will be embedded in delivery of everyday care.

When a strategy goes wrong ...

Many a health or social care strategy gathers dust on the bookshelf because of the following:

- It's not read or understood. Once a strategy is agreed it needs to be seen, read and understood and discussed by the target audience. Careful thought needs to be given to how key messages are communicated to key movers and shakers.

- It's too vague and woolly. A detailed implementation plan with realistic targets and milestones is vital.
- It's too prescriptive. A strategy that is too detailed without sufficient flexibility may not meet local needs and preferences and then fail to be implemented on a wide scale.
- It lacks ownership. It's essential to engage key players including consumers or patients in your strategy development.
- Potential benefits are not appreciated.
- It has not been linked to other (current or expected) business plans or organisational objectives or priorities.
- Unexpected events – such as a new government initiative, which can send your strategy off course. The strategy should be flexible so that you can adapt it to changed circumstances and new priorities.
- It's launched at the wrong time; it may be ahead of its time or, on the other hand, too late. It's perfectly reasonable to develop a strategy and then pause while you wait for the right time for its implementation (e.g. the next commissioning cycle).
- Financial implications. With many competing priorities for scarce health and social care service resources, your strategy should anticipate financial implications and arrange that appropriate resources be secured.
- Frontline staff who are under pressure with their day-to-day work may be disengaged by changes to the services they deliver – that's thrust upon them without a period of consultation and with no opportunity for co-production of the design and mode of delivery of the revised service.
- No one (or the wrong person) is driving the strategy and implementation plan.

So the development of any type of strategy requires commitment and action from your organisation's leadership (and other organisations which it may affect so you are always aiming for integrated care delivery), to give it authority and agency and achieve general support.

Basic planning processes

The right people should start with a basic assessment of where the organisation is currently, what influences it and what factors affect it – as in Figure 9.1. Consider the immediate conditions and factors that influence your organisation, practice or local health economy.

NHS budgets are increasingly restricted. So business plans supporting strategies and linked implementation plans for TECS need to be focused on service developments and improvements that are (likely to be) cost-effective.

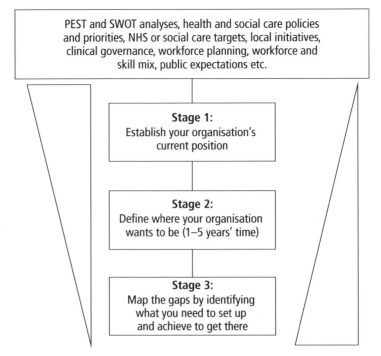

FIGURE 9.1 A simple three-stage model of the planning process

You can use this staged planning process as a substantive activity for a top executive team who is defining their organisation's future purpose for TECS that underpins their strategy and implementation plan. Or adapt it for a directorate or general practice team who wish to plan for delivery via TECS at a team planning meeting.

Environmental perspectives include:

- **p**olitical
- **e**conomical
- **s**ociological
- **t**echnological factors.

Try doing a political, environmental, sociological and technological (PEST) analysis

A PEST analysis (*see* Table 9.1) focuses on factors external to the organisation, allowing analysis of drivers that may or may not be within your organisation's control. Your PEST analysis should be carried out in the context of the broader picture – the 'climate' in which your organisation operates. This will reflect the perspectives and issues of other health and social care providers, patient groups and target population and the current local situation (politically). It should draw on any local profiles, audits and surveys that are relevant and already available.

EXERCISE 9.1   PEST analysis

Discuss the political, economic, sociological and technological factors that influence your organisation's aims and objectives in relation to the creation and effective delivery of TECS with colleagues. Then write up your report as a draft that everyone who has participated can critique, which you then revise and share with others of influence on the service or who will be affected, for their perspectives. Then make further revisions or additions as appropriate.

TABLE 9.1 PEST analysis framework for you to complete

Political	Economic
Sociological	Technological

A strengths weaknesses opportunities threats (SWOT) analysis might be useful too

A SWOT analysis (*see* Table 9.2) allows you to analyse the internal factors that contribute to the current situation within an organisation. Undertaking a SWOT analysis will focus on the internal factors that drive the organisation forward and give it purpose. The analysis will reflect the vision of the organisation, its strategies, objectives and priorities, its functions and its 'rules' of how it engages with other organisations or people. This will include the range of services provided and financial information, costs, cash flow etc.

EXERCISE 9.2 SWOT analysis

Identify internal control factors (strengths and weaknesses) and external control factors (opportunities and threats) that influence you or your organisation's ability to achieve the aims and objectives for the set-up and delivery of TECS. Then share, consult or revise the SWOT analysis as described for Exercise 9.1.

TABLE 9.2 SWOT analysis framework for you to complete

Strengths	Weaknesses
Opportunities	Threats

Implementing your strategy

Stick with your organisation's priorities: working more productively, improving specific clinical management, attaining required outcomes. Find out what technology enabled approaches or equipment there are available to you in your organisation, or within your health or social care role, or accessible to your patients or service users or the general public at large. Then be decisive – challenge the status quo.

Focus your drive and energy on the clinical or health and well-being value of any new mode of digital delivery. Create and adopt effective digital delivery of care that is focused on achieving improved clinical outcomes for patients or service users for whom you are responsible (as well as savings on costs of delivery).

Frontline practitioners who'll be vital supporters of TECS if a new mode of digital care is to be adopted will be positively driven by gaining better clinical outcomes for individual patients and population sub-groups with long-term conditions or poor lifestyle habits; managers will be driven by overall financial savings as well as clinical benefits and better positions on comparison league tables. Keep abreast of what day-to-day challenges anyone involved is experiencing and try to find solutions proactively to keep the adoption and dissemination going.

Focus on likely positive achievements that will drive everyone's enthusiasm and increase support for TECS such as:

- preventing deterioration of a health condition; for example, for people with COPD by triggering them to initiate rescue medication (a short course of antibiotics with or without a course of steroid medication) in line with symptoms and signs pre-agreed in a shared care management plan with their responsible clinician
- enhancing clinical management of a health condition; for example, titrating up or stepping down medication at the right time, such as for worsening heart failure or newly diagnosed hypertension or newly treated Parkinson's disease or where drugs for different conditions clash
- improving clinical productivity and thus releasing time to provide care
- supporting social care; for example, detecting or preventing falls, or encouraging compliance, taking medication via an automated pill dispenser or with associated reminder messages delivered by mobile phone texts
- encouraging improved lifestyle habits; for example, boosting smoking cessation support, sustaining a weight management programme, cutting down excessive alcohol consumption
- stimulating and sustaining behaviour change; for example, complying with prescribed medication or recommended interventions such as regular exercise, avoiding stressors, minimising causes of vascular dementia, such as by pushing a person to quit smoking
- supporting a person's self-care; for example, boosting their confidence in taking responsibility for their health condition, helping them to understand their conditions and thus increasing the likelihood that they invest in self-care
- focusing on a specific purpose; for example, reducing numbers of avoidable hospital admissions or unnecessary face-to-face consultations with GPs or practice teams; reducing frequency of home visits by community nurses
- including all types of patients or service users; for example, older people with complex co-morbidities, those with pressure ulcers, teenagers who are reluctant to attend face-to-face healthcare for review of their established health condition (e.g. asthma, diabetes, depression)
- basing TECS in all kinds of settings; for example, self-care in a person's home, or care provided in general practice, pharmacies, acute hospitals; or community care from district nurse or mental health nurse teams
- providing modes of care that suit a person's needs and preferences in line with available resources: owned or lent equipment (e.g. own mobile phone or sphygmomanometer; or borrowed pulse oximeter) or tool (e.g. self-selected mobile phone app)
- enhancing access and availability to health and social care; for example, via telephone, email, Skype or video consultation with a health or social care professional

- providing health coaching; for example, follow on one-to-one or group interaction via Facebook or telephone interaction or video conferencing.

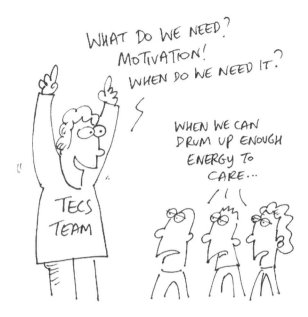

Create a communication plan

Your communication plan should aim to:

- support your organisation in maximising the impact of developing TECS
- provide stakeholders with the knowledge, information, materials or training that they need to use TECS effectively
- ensure that communications about the programmes are open, clear, concise, transparent and timely
- make evidence available to a wide audience, sharing and publishing case studies and using social media – so appealing to different population groups
- engage different groups of the workforce (practitioners, managers, administrators, leads) in various health and social care settings
- use case studies to showcase the impact that TECS can have.

It is crucial to outline the key messages of the communication plan in order for the communication messaging to be targeted accordingly, as in the following examples.

- 'We are committed to using TECS to help patients take responsibility for the monitoring and shared management of their own condition, treatment, and supporting good lifestyle habits.'

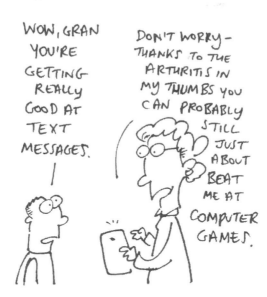

- 'We aim to combine different technologies and ways of working to transform care delivery.'
- 'The information revolution will change the way everyone engages in their own healthcare. This will encourage patients to take responsibility for the management of their health and long-term conditions supported by their clinician or care workers.'
- 'We will encourage those who are sceptical of the use of TECS to modify their views, by sharing knowledge and experience within and across teams with lots of case studies and examples that demonstrate how staff or people benefit from the applications of TECS.'

Evaluation

If your organisation has invested resources and effort in commissioning or setting up and providing TECS for its local population, it will want to know that the investment was worth it. So you'll need to collect data and user perspectives that can be matched against the success criteria or against measures specified in the business plan or strategy that inform the attainment of the organisation's priorities. You might adopt a holistic approach capturing data and users' experiences that pertain to survival, morbidity (physical and psychological), social and family or personal issues. Or you might focus on specific measures relating to best practice clinical outcomes and personal behaviour (e.g. adherence to interventions or medication defined in their care plan).[4]

You'll be aiming to gather evidence that indicates that investing in digital delivery of care detects a person's health problems or initial signs of deterioration earlier, which triggers appropriate patient or service user actions or rapid clinician/carer responses which avoid unnecessary health or social care usage and ultimately saves NHS or social care funds.

Outcomes will range from enhanced patient autonomy to sustained motivation, as follows.

1. Enhanced patient autonomy – understanding their long-term condition better or the adverse effects of poor lifestyle habits; the patient remaining independent at home rather than entering a continuing care home; joint titration of medication or other interventions against an agreed management plan.
2. Change in healthcare usage – hopefully fewer or no avoidable hospital admissions or trips to A&E; more effective medication regimes and less wastage as patients take medication regularly at the right dose and right time; fewer follow-up visits to GP or any other overseeing clinician as remote transmission of patient's vital signs or other bodily measures safely substitute for face-to-face clinic visits, with at least as good quality of care. See www. nuffieldtrust.org.uk/publications/impact-telehealth-use-hospital-care-and-mortality for a recent relevant report on the impact of telehealth.
3. Improved clinical outcomes when a patient's vital signs and test results are available to clinicians caring for them from afar – in real time or close to real time. This enables more rapid titration of medication (e.g. antihypertensive drugs) or initiation of medication to prevent deterioration when telehealth responses indicate an exacerbation of a health condition (e.g. rescue medication for COPD; or step up/step down dose regimes for asthma).
4. Increased patient satisfaction as they have a more positive experience of care, when they or their carer (e.g. family member) are trusted to measure aspects of their health (e.g. home blood pressure readings, oxygen saturation levels, weight) or well-being (e.g. mental health scores) and relay reliable responses to the responsible clinicians.
5. Sustained motivation – to persist with smoking cessation, weight management and alcohol-free lifestyle, through regular encouragement and questioning, so individuals do not give up on tough days.

Read and understand more about the types of evaluation of services, or people's perspectives you can consider using, in Chapter 16.

It can be difficult to obtain reliable data about health or social care usage from the different settings that provide multidisciplinary care to an individual patient or service user. But hopefully the national drive to provide digital, real-time and interoperable patient and care records will help with individuals identified via their unique NHS number. So the health system's wide adoption and optimisation of mobile technologies will enable health and social care professionals, service users and carers to collaborate effectively in the organisation, delivery and evaluation of care in the acute, primary care, community and home care settings.[2,3]

FAQs

Q1. Are there any useful resources for implementation of TECS that you'd recommend?

A. Try these – they give variety across the various types of digital delivery of care:

- Ready, Steady, Go: a telehealth implementation toolkit. National Institute for Health Research. Available at: https://drive.google.com/file/d/0B3-SF4FxenwJQkZOakszb21GRW8/view?pref=2&pli=1
- Assisted Living Technology and Services Learning and Development Framework. Skills for Care. Available at: www.skillsforcare.org.uk/Skills/Assisted-Living-Technologies/Assisted-living-technology.aspx
- Telehealth resources at the Royal College of Nursing. Available at: www2.rcn.org.uk/development/practice/e-health/telehealth_and_telecare
- Skills for Care *Commissioner's Guide*. Available at: http://cat.skillsforcare.org.uk/Commissioners-Guide
- NHS Commissioning Assembly. *Technology Enabled Care Services: resource for commissioners*. London: NHS England; 2015. Available at: www.england.nhs.uk/wp-content/uploads/2015/04/TECS_FinalDraft_0901.pdf

Q2. Is there a good example of a region-wide strategic approach to digital delivery?

A. The West Midlands network and 'get connected' site show the achievement of social care leaders in establishing assistive technology on a wide scale for the people who need and can benefit from telecare. See http://wm-adass.org.uk/thematic-improvement-networks/west-midlands-connected/

References

1. NHS Commissioning Assembly. *Technology Enabled Care Services: resource for commissioners*. London: NHSE; 2015. Available at: www.england.nhs.uk/wp-content/uploads/2015/04/TECS_FinalDraft_0901.pdf
2. NHS National Information Board. *Personalised Health and Care 2020: using data and technology to transform outcomes for patients and citizens; a framework for action*. London: HM Government; 2014. Available at: www.gov.uk/government/uploads/system/uploads/attachment_data/file/384650/NIB_Report.pdf
3. NHS National Information Board. *National Information Board's Workstream Roadmaps*. London: NHS National Information Board; 2015. Available at: www.gov.uk/government/publications/national-information-boards-workstream-roadmaps
4. Health Foundation. *Evaluation: what to consider*. London: Health Foundation; 2015. Available at: www.health.org.uk/sites/default/files/EvaluationWhatToConsider.pdf

Chapter 10

Making digital delivery happen as an individual manager or practitioner: adopting established technology and innovation

Dr Ruth Chambers

Innovation should be everyone's business – whether that is inventing a better way of doing things and making a difference to people's lives, or adopting a great new way of delivering care that has been established elsewhere as being worthwhile, or contributing to local dissemination. Remember that technology is an enabler of effective delivery of health or social care and not the solution or prescribed treatment or intervention. It might help the person take more responsibility for their health, or aid a health or social care professional to track a person's progress for the likes of wound care or clinical control of their long-term condition.

Taking forward innovation

The development, implementation and spread of innovation are central to the commissioning of service redesign and service improvement. All innovative initiatives or interventions should be evaluated to determine whether they are successful before rolling out or proportionately decommissioning or disinvesting in products or services that the innovative idea, service or product replaces or improves.

There are three levels of innovation (*see* Figure 10.1). Level 1 innovations may involve transfer of a product or service to health or social care from another service or industry, or be genuinely novel. Level 2 innovations will already have been tried in some healthcare context (may be outside the UK), in a different setting or for another purpose than the one proposed. Level 3 innovations have already been tried locally or elsewhere but need adapting or refining.[1,2]

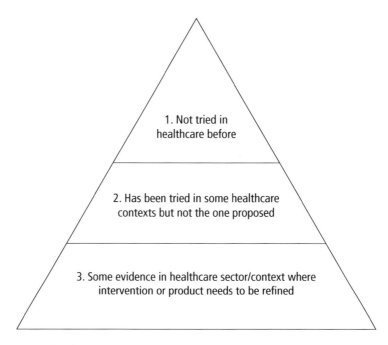

FIGURE 10.1 Levels of innovation

Investment of funding and effort in innovation should be targeted at the following.[3]

- The organisation's strategic vision: putting patients, carers and the public first; ensuring consistent high-quality healthcare; health outcomes; operating with minimum bureaucracy; delivering best value for money.
- Your organisation's priorities; for example, (re)admission avoidance; interventions that optimise the capacity and capability of the workforce.

NHS and local authority organisations should seek out the latest evidence for research and innovations to feed routinely into the design and provision of local services. They should utilise innovation to reduce unwarranted variation and drive greater compliance with NICE guidance – in service design and provision of care, and training and education of managers and clinicians. This information and evidence should then be used in associated business plans to justify the proposed investment.

Areas of focus for innovation

Possible areas of focus for innovation that should be worth investing money, time and effort in include:

- redesign of primary care (or other care setting) services
- enhanced quality and safety
- integrated working across health and care settings
- new or adapted technology for different purposes
- improving capacity and efficiency.

You as an innovator?

So you might lead on this innovation in your workplace or support others or your own team. You might even try to change the way that an element of health or social care is delivered in a large organisation (e.g. a hospital or community nursing service or a general practice or federation of practices) in a system-wide way that is focused on a clinical pathway or defined population. If you opt for a type of technology on your own and operate it in a solo manner it might disrupt your team or not be as effectual as it would be if delivered by a group of professionals or adopted on a wide scale across your organisation or local health economy as part of a technology enabled care services (TECS) strategy and implementation plan.

EXERCISE 10.1   How do you fare as an innovator?

Have a go at analysing your strengths by completing Table 10.1; then discuss your perspectives with others who know how you perform at work.

TABLE 10.1 Self-rating of the basic skills that you need as an effective innovator

Are you good at …?	Yes	No
Overcoming barriers		
Providing evidence of the positive values of your selected innovation		
Being persistent to make something happen		
Leading – people, service change		
Recognising your own and others' skills – and utilising them		
Obtaining resources to enable innovation development and dissemination		

Build on your skills and passion to make change happen:

Don't be afraid of barriers: believe that if you persist in taking forward your idea or early stage of your project that you can overcome these barriers and make that innovation succeed. You need to recognise what the likely barriers are and understand them. You won't be able to ride roughshod over them as you might breach national regulations or run out of resources or cause antagonism that blocks your progress or the adoption of your innovative mode of delivery.

Celebrate the successes of innovations that work and learn from your or others' projects or pilots that don't work out. Write up your progress and success, sharing the **evidence** of what the innovation is or what it has achieved and get that published on websites, as articles in journals or newsletters, tweet about it, talk about it or go online – locally or nationally to all relevant types of audiences. You can combine targeting health or social care professionals or managers or go directly to patients and the general public in your communications plan. That means that you should be planning and gathering evidence at the baseline (including if relevant and possible, indicators or benchmarking of provision of care for 12 months or so before baseline) and throughout the delivery of the innovation. That might be from users' or professionals' perspectives or impartial measurements of progress, such as bodily measurements such as weight, blood pressure, or clinical and other local or national indicators or outcomes such as healthcare usage or public health-related achievements.

Be self-disciplined and persistent in taking forward a well-justified (well, according to your thinking anyway!) innovation; but don't be (too) disruptive. You need to believe in yourself – and recognise that it often takes much longer to move from the idea to an actual product or process or mode of delivery than you'd previously anticipated; and progress from a local application to use on a wide scale by many people or organisations. Give your project enough time to succeed. Anticipate and overcome the blocks – with good leadership, better infrastructure and dedicated resources, by actually changing the culture of professionals and patients or general public, and moving to more supportive organisational management. Be decisive; be proud of your tenacity. Go for positive disruption to make constructive change happen if you're working in a 'same old, same old' culture where people talk a great deal about change in inactive ways. Don't wreck the good elements of your service delivery, engage well at all levels, focus on organisational priorities – and persist with service improvements. Regard self-discipline as learnt behaviour – which you'll continue to strengthen through your own reflections and positive feedback from others.

Try to be an inspirational leader: communicate your compelling vision of a new way of working. You need an achievable vision about which everyone can appreciate the potential – to increase productivity, provide more convenient health or social care services, enhance the quality of services within budget or without any extra costs or even with obvious savings with associated reinvestment. Your vision should match others' priorities if you want them to support you and increase the likelihood of speeding to your goals. Your success is **moving along** the path to your goals, not just actually getting there with others adopting the product or process you are promoting or providing. You will likely have to influence or guide systematic change and either lead that change or stimulate others to do so, such as by creating or supporting pressure groups. Resist the temptation to become boastful or complacent or intolerant of dissent. Stay focused and use your willpower and self-discipline to continue striving to achieve your goals.

Work with people with the right skill mix to develop and roll out this innovation: the person who invents something is usually a different sort of person and thinker from those who focus on the development of applications and put them into practice or engage others to do so. An inventor would not usually have the experience or skills or be in the right role to draft the organisational strategy, consult on it or get sign-up and budget, and roll out with associated upskilling and problem solving. Work with the commissioning and care delivery teams in flexible ways. Engage with expected end users to ensure that the product or process meets their needs and preferences; redesign it if it doesn't – be humble about your idea and vision and be prepared to modify your innovation as the end user usually knows best. Ensure that clinical safety is prioritised, your evidence of safety and benefits is valid and is implemented in your digital delivery programme.

Find those resources that you need to make the innovation happen. You can't just make innovation happen in your spare time. Yes, you are likely to be motivated by drivers to improve quality; but to develop and sell the potential benefits of the innovation to others so that they buy it, adopt it or disseminate it, show that you have saved on costs. 'Invest to save' has been a mantra in the NHS and social care for a long time – and still is – at least in theory as there's often minimal evidence of this when innovations are launched and consequence costs have not been envisaged or allowed for. So learn to write a business case that focuses on achieving the goals in a time frame and manner that the potential funder will rate as vital if they are to agree the funds that you need to complete the pilot and rollout.

So you need to understand about risk management, for instance, or work with someone who does – risk stratification of patient groups will help you to target your innovation to optimise benefits for investment. And to be really successful in achieving widespread adoption and dissemination you need to anticipate the barriers that will crop up, already have identified resources to combat them (maybe money, training programmes, support groups) and to meet (or better still avoid) consequence costs (e.g. if your favoured mode of digital delivery relies on costly specialised practitioners to respond with face-to-face meetings pretty often if they distrust remote delivery of care).

Build or renew your personal development plan so that you have reserved time and resources to learn new skills or seek different experiences as needed if you are to be effective in your role or are building your expertise for the future. You'll need the support of your line manager if you're in an employee position or maybe a senior colleague.

You need good project planning to move from planning to implementation, from the pilot phase to widespread dissemination across the workforce or population or sub-groups. You need to support the transition from existing delivery of care to the improved service or practice which is more effective or productive or meets people's needs and preferences in enabling ways that trigger their behavioural change.

Invest in communication: you must engage with everyone relevant to the innovation – funding it, adopting it, receiving it (patients and service users) or learning from it (health or social care professionals; managers; patients or the general public). Manage people's expectations – yes, you are talking your innovation up, but be realistic too (from their perspectives) with a positive theme.

Invest in training. Don't be afraid to admit that you are unsure about using technology. The market is moving so quickly that the system struggles to keep up with the latest innovations. If you are serious about using technology to improve services, familiarise yourself with the market. Whether this is training or research, learning from others will make the job of transforming services much easier.

Tolerate risk and challenges: there is a great deal of interest from the NHS and social care about ways to provide more effective care – but much nervousness about investing in new products and systems, especially if the opportunities are not evidence based. We need continual medical and social innovation – with a cycle that moves along to implementation in smooth, synchronised ways. That means a national cultural change for commissioners and providers of health and social care – which innovative individuals can help drive. You should continually anticipate and minimise the likelihood of risk. Plan and adopt parallel actions to mitigate such risks if they do happen. Little will happen if you just think about an innovation and don't act. Work though conflict promptly and fairly, letting everyone know where they stand. Think through complex problems and gauge the meaning from whatever data and information is available, adding your personal experience as you interpret the situation and drive forward plans.

Work with practitioners who'll benefit from digital modes of delivery: that's frontline practitioners as well as clinical directors and leads as you devise the scope and content and applications of the digital content. You will need to overcome professional inertia – many health or social care professionals are 'allergic' to innovation and avoid it, making excuses and exaggerating any inconvenience from this potential change in service delivery. Listen to frontline workers' ideas and suggestions – don't be hierarchical about how an innovation should be adopted or rolled out; adapt your implementation plan for any particular setting or purpose or practitioner preferences, as far as that is appropriate and feasible.

Work with patients and carers who'll benefit from the digital mode of delivery: you'll need to convince individual patients or their carers that they can take more control over their life (they may not believe this). You'll need to show people how technology really can make a difference. Consider whether and when interactivity is better, or when information can just be pushed at the person receiving digital care – and make a difference to their beliefs or behaviour. Gauge what inconvenience they will tolerate for the benefits they'll accrue – on a pain versus pleasure balance. Many individuals are not used to looking after themselves, for example, by taking personal responsibility for their lifestyle habits or clinical management, so it won't come automatically to them to look after their long-term conditions. Don't forget that a person themselves may initiate digital care through their chosen app that they have obtained or purchased. Their health or social care practitioner then needs to be prepared to include this in their care management if the information and messaging are trustworthy.

Demonstrate improved health outcomes through the solutions you are providing via digital modes of delivery. Future users want to see the evidence of benefits or frequency of any adverse events and how any new programme meets users' needs and preferences – whether that of health or social care users or patient/carer users. So your various types of evaluation will need to cover clinical, technical and functional elements of the digital modes of delivery or programme, and meet the needs and expectations of commissioners and providers by, for example, providing evidence of impact and potential savings in the business case.

EXAMPLE 10.1 Inventor Phil O'Connell MBCS CITP

Phil is the creator of the NHS's patented simple telehealth technology, methodology and Florence (or Flo) – the mobile phone simple texting programme. Phil invented Flo with and for the NHS as a pioneering, ultra-low-cost, massively scalable and multi award-winning telehealth solution and is responsible for taking this ground-breaking innovation from concept to large-scale deployment across the NHS.

Phil is a chartered IT professional specialising in organisational, process and business change. Phil has a wealth of NHS telehealth and commercial sector experience from senior roles across Europe, Russia, Africa and the South Pacific in the pharmaceutical, telecommunications, software and consulting sectors. He is a visiting fellow at Staffordshire University and honorary lecturer at Keele University. Phil has won NHS Leadership Academy accolades of The NHS Innovator of the Year (2012) and The NHS Inspirational Leader of the Year (2013). He also works as a clinical messaging consultant to the US Department of Veterans Affairs.

Take account of regulatory powers: be decisive, bold in your vision and forward planning for how you might create a digital delivery programme or service – but be aware of the regulations that are relevant to the digital modes of delivery, relating to patient confidentiality, data sharing and the like. Search for and understand professional codes of performance where social media or technology enabled services feature. Be sensitive to regulatory powers and fit in with their scope and guidance; for example, that a diagnostic component of digital delivery will mean that the digital equipment is classified as a 'medical device'.

Understanding how to make change happen

Figure 10.2 describes the stages in the cycle of change through which an individual moves and how they must be motivated to change. So potential individual users pass through the stage of contemplation (e.g. use of a different method of delivery of healthcare such as Skype) and on to the stage of taking action for themselves. They need realistic targets for that change that are achievable so as not to demotivate them or allow them an escape route ('I knew I couldn't do it.'). In this case the cycle of change, as applied to the use of Skype between patient and clinician, needs to be populated with different actions or approaches for the individual patient and practitioner, but it is the same progression around the cycle with support and an experience that maintains that change.

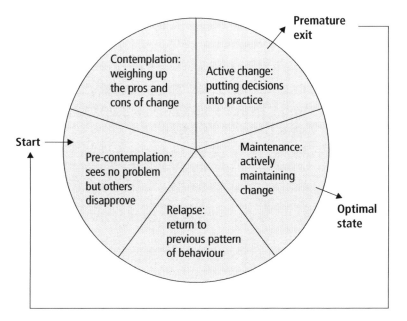

FIGURE 10.2 Cycle of change

To understand what intervention to use to try to help people to change, you need to determine whether individuals are ready to change or have already taken action. Then you can match your approach or intervention to the stage at which they are.

The five stages of change illustrated in Figure 10.2 include the following.[4]

1. Pre-contemplation: 'the stage at which there is no intention to change behaviour in the foreseeable future'.
2. Contemplation: 'the stage in which people are aware that a problem exists and are seriously thinking about overcoming it but have not yet made a commitment to take action'.
3. Preparation: 'the stage that combines intention and behavioural criteria.

Individuals in this stage are intending to take action in the next month and (may) have unsuccessfully taken action in the past year'.

4. Action: 'the stage in which individuals modify their behaviour, experiences, or environment in order to overcome their problems'.
5. Maintenance: 'the stage in which people work to prevent relapse and consolidate the gains attained during the action'.

Individuals who refuse to engage with change, such as new ways of delivering care, may:

- be generally passive
- find challenge frightening and avoid it whenever possible
- avoid seeking insight into themselves and their beliefs
- find feedback and criticism threatening
- have low reserves of energy
- have poor motivation
- resent others' success
- fail to realise their potential.

Sometimes the resistance to change arises from a malfunctioning organisation or practice team such as:

- poor management of quality processes
- inadequate infrastructure and insufficient resources to undertake tasks
- poor communication within the work setting
- an unhealthy culture within the organisation
- a culture of fear and lack of openness among practitioners and managers
- inappropriate styles of management and organisational structure.

Clinicians who see the need and potential benefit of using TECS should be willing to select appropriate patients, interact effectively with individual patients and undertake proactive management. Easily accessible support will be required for health or social care teams while they familiarise themselves with the system or mode of delivery, associated documentation and strategies to engage and monitor successful users of the new system. To prevent disengagement of clinicians or social workers through frustration, irritation or perceptions of the TECS being difficult to implement, protocols need to be easily and widely adaptable to ensure that they are tailored to individual users' needs and the exact problem on which the service delivery method is focused.

And, lastly, to make your innovation happen:

- have courage
- be open minded, reflect, rethink
- collaborate and swap or share ideas – develop a shared vision

- find investment – from industry, academia, commissioners, providers (matching their strategies or priorities); make the most of opportunities
- don't give up!

FAQs

Q1. There are many innovators about but not all are successful. What areas should I focus on in the NHS where I would be most likely to succeed?

A. Focus on 'low hanging fruit' such as long-term conditions where more effective self-care or earlier prevention in social or healthcare, or shared management along the pathway(s), can minimise or avoid deterioration which in turn reduces healthcare usage, such as with:

- heart failure
- atrial fibrillation
- asthma
- COPD
- neurodegeneration (e.g. dementia)
- cancer
- falls
- adverse lifestyle habits.

These are the health conditions or lifestyle behaviours that crush our health and social care economies where we do too little proactively for the huge numbers of people with these conditions or who have self-abusive lifestyle habits. So focus on associated preventive ways or providing optimal treatment or engaging with people with these conditions and motivating them to change their behaviour. Health and social care economic crises are looming with the increasing proportion of older people and rising prevalence rates of long-term conditions. So we need more innovations in digital delivery of care that enhance efficiencies. We need to complete the innovation cycle from invention, to early adopters to widespread dissemination of the innovation and maybe commercialisation of the products – to sell such assets abroad maybe.

Q2. How safe is it to transfer responsibility to a patient or service user to look after their own health and well-being – especially if they've got early dementia or are in a depressed state?

A. Take an intelligent view of a person's safety: you can share responsibility for TECS with the user – so you are not their safety 'marshal' night and day – you have to learn to delegate and trust the patient or service user to stick to the pre-agreed shared care management plan. Digital delivery of care is about empowering the patient or service user, so a health or social care professional must guide the user and then step back, providing ongoing oversight. This is your opportunity to agree a care plan with reliable information and guidance for the patient or service user to follow in informed ways. The care professional will need to judge their cognitive ability and mental state as well as their willingness when they assess the patient or service user for the type or mode of digital delivery and agree a particular care management plan with them. But it is likely that without this resource or the TECS application, the patient or service user will seek alternative sources to update them on their condition and then follow other unreliable paths for their care.

References

1. Health Foundation. *SHINE 2012: call for proposals*. London: Health Foundation; 2012. (Derived from their 4 Levels of Innovation.)
2. Health Foundation. *Evaluation: what to consider*. London: Health Foundation; 2015. Available at: www.health.org.uk/sites/default/files/EvaluationWhatToConsider.pdf
3. Department of Health (DH). *Innovation Health and Wealth: accelerating adoption and diffusion in the NHS*. London: DH; 2011. Available at: www.institute.nhs.uk/images/documents/Innovation/Innovation%20Health%20and%20Wealth%20-%20accelerating%20adoption%20and%20diffusion%20in%20the%20NHS.pdf
4. Chambers R. Getting organised for supporting self care as an individual professional in the general practice team. In: Chambers R, Wakley G, Blenkinsopp A. *Supporting Self Care in Primary Care*. Abingdon: Radcliffe Publishing; 2006. pp. 30–42.

Chapter 11

Commissioning, implementing and mainstreaming technology enabled care services

Jayne Birch-Jones

Commission for outcomes, not for technology

Technology enabled care services (TECS) should be built into the commissioning culture in the NHS to become a standard stream within any long-term condition care pathway to deliver better outcomes and support integration and collaboration between health and social care services and other providers. But any such pathway should allow for local flexibility and adaptation.

But commissioners don't know everything. So they need independent support for service redesign and the associated decommissioning of services already in place.

Technology should be seen as an enabler for improvement of health and social care services. However, too often there is a focus on commissioning technology rather than delivery. The health and social care workforce should be supported to make TECS a normal part of the assessment and care planning. We need to deliver paper-light services in the NHS and social care to support their long-term sustainability. This is a real challenge, but one which should generate substantial cost savings – NHS England projects potential cost savings of up to £10 billion by 2020 over a five-year dissemination and adoption period for evolving TECS. There are restrictions that can be easily overcome to turn projections into reality, such as making Wi-Fi freely available in all NHS settings so enabling clinicians and care staff to use hand-held devices in their everyday work and creating a 'paperless' service.

Evolution of TECS

In December 2011, the English Government published its *Life Sciences Prospectus*[1] which identified the most appropriate medical innovation developments for manufacture and uptake with the potential to save £1.2 billion a year and boost clinical effectiveness. This included high-impact technologies such as telehealth intended for accelerated adoption by the NHS.

The Whole Systems Demonstrator (WSD) programme was set up as the world's largest randomised control trial to evaluate benefits and effectiveness of telehealth and telecare services.[2] It measured the impact of telehealth on reducing hospital admissions and patient mortality rates. The Nuffield Trust recommended that NHS and social care commissioners 'concentrate on service redesign, craft incentives, tackle entrenched practices, use data intelligently, try telehealth soberly as part of a wider set of changes and evaluate as you go' and involve clinicians and patients in targeting TECS to generate better value.[3]

EXAMPLE 11.1   A whole systems approach to establishing TECS across health and social care sectors in Nottinghamshire

The main body of this chapter is presented as a case study that describes the experience and lessons learned of the whole system approach taken across Nottinghamshire in implementing a TECS programme across the health and social care community. This starts by relaying the four background activities.

1. Clinical event: identified need to use assistive technology (AT) to support clinical care delivery

Nottinghamshire clinical commissioning groups (CCGs) and providers of health and social care (i.e. NHS trusts and the local authority) established a collaborative programme of work to create efficiencies as quality, innovation, partnership and productivity (QIPP) savings. The programme was called Productive Notts. A clinical stakeholder event was held in January 2011 where telehealth or care was identified as a priority area which was projected to yield significant benefits in terms of quality of care and improved use of clinical resources.

2. Team appointed

An AT workstream was established to take forward the recommendations made at the stakeholder event. The chief officer of two of the CCGs was appointed executive lead to take overall responsibility for delivery with a GP to provide clinical leadership.

A budget was identified and a three month timescale agreed to create a business case to be submitted to the executive team.

A programme manager was employed initially for three months to develop the business case; they had a clinical background as well as information management and technology (IM&T) programme management experience including the creation of business cases.

3. Literature review, patient views and baseline captured

To ground the business case on good evidence and focus on the requirements of the local health and social care community, several background activities were undertaken:

- a literature review to identify telehealth or care research and good practice from other areas of the NHS and social care – what works and what doesn't. This identified that telehealth was commonly used for COPD. The review concluded that patient inclusion and exclusion criteria in TECS are key to successful implementation to minimise risks of harm, that a range of technology is required to deal with the spectrum of need and that 'one size does not fit all'. Recurring expert opinion from the review identified that telehealth can provide productivity gains and increased quality of care. Cost modelling and benefits analysis were seen to be essential prerequisites to any decisions on investment and implementation, to take into account consequence costs and ensure that there was at least a cost-neutral predicted outcome
- a scoping exercise to identify current AT across Nottinghamshire's local health and social care services. Significant operational use of AT was found to be already in place across health and social care, including video conferencing, telemedicine, telecare and lifestyle monitoring. The community trust provider had recently completed a year's trial of telehealth, but the evaluation report was not available. Nottingham County Council had an AT strategy and Nottingham City CCG and City Council had developed a joint strategy, Better Health and Well Being with Assistive Living Technology, with an associated implementation plan that was being developed. A joint CCG/local authority project manager was in the process of being recruited to take this forward
- patient and public views regarding telehealth care were sought. Patients identified long-term conditions, weight management, epilepsy, arthritis, minor renal problems, glaucoma, smoking cessation, contraception and drugs and alcohol as potential health issues where telehealth could be utilised. Benefits envisaged included fewer visits to the hospital and GP surgery, thus reducing travel and car parking costs; being more convenient; with regular monitoring, continuous record keeping and quicker response times from health or social care professionals.

4. Stakeholder accelerated design event

The fourth background activity undertaken was an accelerated design event (ADE) which brought together key stakeholders in Nottinghamshire to explore research and good practice through presentations and then to identify how telehealth care should be progressed locally.

The purpose of the ADE event was to discuss how the use of telehealth and telecare in Nottinghamshire could support patients with health and social care needs to live more independently, given the backdrop of the local economic and demographic challenges envisaged to be facing Nottinghamshire over the coming years.

The event, which was run with support from the NHS Institute, aimed to answer the question 'How can telehealth care support your care delivery?' The event was based on the 'scan, focus, act' model. During the 'scan' sessions, patients and clinical, social care, managerial and commissioning staff heard about different telehealth and telecare systems by attending several short 'speed dating' presentations. The 'focus' session saw attendees excitedly sharing their views of the presentations and deciding what was felt to be the most appropriate approach for Nottinghamshire. During the final 'act' session, individuals made 60-day pledges in terms of how they would help to implement and drive actions to progress the agreed way forward for telehealth care in Nottinghamshire. These pledges underpinned regular contact with attendees after the event, who were then instrumental in helping to implement telehealth or care across the county so that the first patient was enrolled onto the new telehealth programme within six months of this event.

One of the outputs of the event was the thinking as to how the implementation of telehealth care could contribute to addressing the economic challenges presented. The top priority put forward was to write a business case for implementing a low-cost telehealth system ('Flo', a low-cost simple telehealth solution which, combined with the use of a mobile phone, enables people to manage their conditions from their homes; used widely for enhancing patient self-management, quality of life and providing productivity gains) which was presented at the event, which has been developed by the NHS for the NHS. As well as winning many national awards, this system had been well evaluated and shown to increase patient self-management and quality of life, as well as making the best use of clinical time and financial resources. Around 150 different clinical protocols were on offer, including those for smoking cessation, mental health, hypertension, diabetes, arthritis, asthma, COPD, heart failure, medication compliance, cancer, pulmonary rehabilitation, obstetrics and palliative care.

5. Business case development

The outputs of the literature search, patients' views, baseline of AT local activity and outputs of the ADE were used to create the business case. This was evidence based, focused on the needs of the local population, linked into local as well as national strategies and business plans with buy-in from all key stakeholders. The focus was on implementation of telehealth or care across Nottinghamshire county, to generate improvement in quality of patient care and self-management, productivity gains and cost efficiencies, and avoidance of unnecessary health or social care usage.

6. Clinical workshop held and expressions of interest requested

Another priority was to engage with clinicians and patients to ensure that telehealth or care was driven by care deliverers and service users. A clinical workshop for GPs and specialist nurses from all CCGs in Nottinghamshire was held to demonstrate and discuss the use of Flo simple telehealth in more detail. CCG clinical representatives strongly supported the implementation of Flo. In order to capture the views of GPs and specialist nurses who were unable to attend, a virtual consultation process was undertaken with all clinical stakeholders. Conclusions from this were fed back at each CCG-protected learning event or practice forum, which resulted in gaining delegates' sign-up to progress the use of Flo in cohorts identified by clinicians. Discussions with social care colleagues also took place to identify priority areas for application.

Wider stakeholder events were held to ensure that implementation plans going forward were clinically led; addressed the requirements of patients, clinicians and services; and were incorporated into other service improvements. This was also an opportunity to work towards a single AT strategic plan, taking account of existing telehealth and telecare strategic plans, projects and operational activity within Nottinghamshire, which encouraged organisations to learn from each other, and share experiences, expertise and scarce resources, and reduce duplication of effort.

The enthusiasm and interest of the GPs and other clinicians was unprecedented, with an overwhelming request for demonstrations, which translated into significant numbers of implementations in general practices and other health settings.

7. Business case accepted

The business case was presented and approved in August 2012 with a programme of work up to the end of March 2013, including:

- implementation of simple telehealth care technology and roll out to patient cohorts prioritised by local health community clinicians
- development of a full business case for 2013/14 for further deployment of AT within the Nottinghamshire health and social care community, supporting the community's integrated business plans for 2013/14.

8. Programme progressed

Clinical safety assessment: a full clinical safety assessment was undertaken in line with the then NHS Connecting for Health (CFH) guidelines (now superseded by the Health and Social Care Information Centre ISB 0160 compliance assessment). This was signed off by the CCG's clinical safety officer.

Equipment procured: funded biometric equipment was procured in line with local guidelines following advice on specific equipment from other organisations using the telehealth system. The chosen supplier was a local company that was able to provide a delivery service.

First 'go live' rollout: a heart failure nursing service was the first team to express interest in using Flo simple telehealth as part of its care delivery. Following the development of a simple project plan including some key outcome measures, creation and testing of protocols based on clinical requirements and a short training session, the team went live in November 2012. Clinical staff expressed surprise at the ease of setting up Flo and the speed of enrolment of patients or service users.

Ongoing usage: within three months of 'go live' the Flo programme was producing high levels of patient satisfaction and reductions in their anxiety levels. It provided clear productivity gains for staff by reducing the frequency of home visits and increased monitoring information allowing staff to react quickly to changes in a patient's condition. One clinician reported that using Flo had avoided a hospital admission and reduced the need for extra visits following a clinical exacerbation.

Wider engagement at all levels: there was a significant amount of engagement with other services and teams by the programme manager and clinical lead. Presentations and demonstrations were provided to a plethora of staff at various levels within the organisations, from clinical cabinet and executive meetings to individual service team meetings. As well as undertaking a proactive mapping exercise to identify which services to engage with, requests were received for demonstrations from staff via word of mouth. These began to link into service reviews and development and redesign meetings, as staff began to understand the benefits of Flo, in particular how its use could help address capacity challenges and improve patient self-care.

Additional resource requirements: funded through the business case, a project manager was seconded into the programme to support the increasing engagement activities and further implementation. The project manager was selected for her skills and experience in clinical engagement, change management, project management and knowledge of the local health community. This appointment was key to being able to accelerate 'go lives' with new teams.

First learning event: as a result of feedback from clinicians that while the benefits of utilising Flo were very clear, they sometimes struggled to identify appropriate patients, a half-day event for current and imminent Flo users was organised, to share learning and experiences. This helped to share experiences and consider where implementation might be improved and progressed locally. The need for as much data and evidence as possible to evaluate the outcomes of Flo was highlighted.

Local case studies were presented by clinicians, including a COPD nurse who highlighted why her team started using Flo and what benefits and outcomes the team was hoping to achieve. She also emphasised the simple approach to Flo and how patients seemed to be coping well so far. The heart failure team shared its experiences, highlighting the need to select patients carefully and providing feedback that patients felt reassured using Flo. A patient story was presented about Flo medication reminders and just how something so simple can have an impact on a patient and support them to manage their care needs. Another case study described reduced numbers of consultations by patients who no longer needed to attend a mental health clinic in person.

The clinical lead facilitated a short workshop as to how using telehealth was supporting the QIPP challenge. This feedback was used in the subsequent business case.

Patient engagement: in addition to engaging with clinicians and social care colleagues, the team contacted local patient groups, voluntary, charity and self-care groups including Breathe Easy and Diabetes UK to offer to attend meetings to discuss Flo. This engagement was very successful and resulted in patients proactively discussing their use of Flo with their GP or nurse. Where patients found that their practice was not yet using Flo, patients had been given information to inform their practice about who to contact to get started.

The team also made use of national campaigns such as the national Self Help Week, 'Stoptober', and local events such as annual general meetings to promote the use of telehealth.

Patients using Flo who reported particularly positive and powerful stories about using Flo were asked if they would be willing to share their experiences through the development of case studies to use to demonstrate benefits when engaging with clinicians. The team also worked with internal and external media, radio and television to develop articles and films. Social media was also used to promote good news stories. One patient in particular emerged as a patient champion and has committed significant time to working with the team both locally and nationally. Read more about Josh and how the use of Flo has improved the control of his diabetes in Chapter 8.

9. Justifying subsequent business case based on initial outcomes

A second business case was developed to fund the further implementation of the Flo telehealth programme and to capture evaluation data to support the evidence base that usage was clinically effective and cost-effective and improved the quality and convenience of patient care.

The case for change within the business case was based on feedback from clinicians and patients. Through initial usage, it had been identified that telehealth did help with managing service demand and supporting service redesign. The system was so flexible that it could be used across the whole patient pathway; it seemed simple and low cost and could be quickly implemented. Early evidence showed that the telehealth programme increased patient self-management and their quality of care and led to productivity gains across the services. For instance, using Flo simple telehealth with a cohort of 16 patients with heart failure over an initial three-month period had reduced nurse home visits by a third and prevented one unplanned hospital admission; and patient satisfaction was high.

Other rationales used for the business case were as follows.

- There was a national expectation that CCGs would promote the benefits of technology in improving outcomes, with a particular emphasis on much more rapid take-up of telehealth and telecare in line with patient need.
- A new Direct Enhanced Service for general practice teams designed to provide remote care monitoring for patients with long-term conditions would incentivise general practice teams to initiate and adopt TECS.

- Increased use of telehealth was one of the qualifying targets for the Commissioning for Quality and Innovation (CQUIN) 2013/14 for provider NHS trusts.
- The Department of Health (DH) highlighted that at least 3 million people in England with long-term conditions and/or social care needs could benefit from the use of telehealth and telecare services; for Nottinghamshire, this figure equated to 60 000 people.[2]
- Clinical engagement with Flo had been very positive and staff had been very proactive in identifying innovative ways to use Flo.

The business case aimed to have 250 patients enrolled onto Flo across Nottinghamshire by the end of March 2013.

Nottinghamshire was establishing a national reputation for its excellent telehealth clinical engagement which was recognised at DH level. This resulted in a flood of contacts from other NHS organisations asking for information and guidance support. The programme manager was part of the NHS England/US Department of Veterans Affairs (VA) mobile health partnership scheme, which exchanges learning and best practice between the UK and USA. The local health and social care community became involved in a national rollout of Flo telehealth, which provided some matched funding and access to eight nationally developed clinical protocols (covering several long-term conditions and medication reminders), which were mapped to the five domains of the NHS Outcomes Framework.[4] The pledge was for at least 1000 additional patients to be enrolled onto Flo across Nottinghamshire in 2013/14, adding to the 250 patients expected to be signed up by the end of March 2013. These cohorts formed the basis of the business case.

The work stream along with commissioning, contracting and frontline health and social care staff were involved in scoping the likely areas for telehealth implementation over the following year. They included a wide range of TECS products in addition to Flo in their review, which could provide support for patients with more complex care requirements. However, without exception, these alternative technology products were significantly more expensive, required clinical monitoring or a call centre-type approach to manage breaches of pre-set thresholds, and did not in most cases have clearly identified benefits and cost-effectiveness data.

The business case was approved by the Nottinghamshire Executive Team (Nottinghamshire-wide chief officers). This provided the approved budget for a further year and included extra funding for a part-time support officer to help with the significant volume of training and demonstrations. This post was filled by a member of staff from the local community who had significant experience as a GP system trainer, bringing with her significant knowledge and connections in the local primary care community. This helped significantly with the continuing effective engagement with health and social care professionals.

10. Usage of telehealth written into provider contracts, clinical strategies and business plans

The conditions of the business case approval included the incorporation of telehealth being factored in to provider contract negotiations and seen as a net benefit when calculating growth requirements. The thinking behind this was that the use of TECS would help the providers to deal with increasing demand from service users within the same cost base.

The team engaged with CCG contracting staff to enhance members' understanding of TECS and provide support during contract negotiations. As organisations had already started to write the use of Flo into their clinical strategies and business plans, the incorporation within contracts was straightforward and the detail in relation to specific usage was available.

The service was also a key enabler to the Mid Nottinghamshire's 'Better Together' transformation programme which encouraged integrated primary and acute care systems (PACS).

11. Spreading local experience at regional and national levels

The programme manager was asked to provide some operational support to the national clinical rollout of the Advice and Interactive Messaging (AIM) for Health[5] project as an acknowledgement of the best practice and success of the use of Flo in Nottinghamshire.

This was a mutually beneficial arrangement, with Nottinghamshire good practice being shared with other organisations, in particular those who were finding clinical engagement challenging. For Nottinghamshire, it provided an income source to fund a wider rollout.

The East Midlands Academic Health Science Network (EMAHSN) provided support and funding for the evaluation; local work stream staff had engaged with the EMAHSN to discuss and identify best practice in terms of speeding up adoption. One of the areas that the team found particularly challenging in terms of support needed was with the acute provider trusts. Advice was sought from the EMAHSN in relation to how to address this; a business case was approved to fund a fixed-term clinical project manager to provide Nottinghamshire acute hospitals with dedicated resources to implement TECS. The post has been extended for a further year and TECS have become embedded into services.

12. Evaluation of initial pilots

Evaluation data collated from user teams and all patients using Flo was analysed and findings written up by an independent evaluator.

A simple two-part questionnaire was included in each patient pack with a return envelope to their clinician. The patient received a reminder to complete the qualitative section of the questionnaire via texted responses to Flo. The clinician also completed a question set for that patient. In addition providers identified the number of GP appointments, A&E attendances and hospital admissions each patient had prior to, and post, use of Flo. The findings were limited by patient recruitment numbers, but identified significant quality, cost and clinical benefits to patients using Flo.

Successive annual evaluations have been undertaken; each time with an increased number of patients and quantity of data collected and with differing emphases on patient cohorts.

13. 2014/15 business case developed: increased numbers engaged and Flo operationalised

Throughout 2013/14, the use and applications of Flo increased and patient and staff engagement continued to be very positive; it appeared that Flo had gone viral across Nottinghamshire! The resulting figures in March 2014 were in excess of 2400 patients signed up to Flo.

Given that its use was now entering its third year, it was agreed with the executive lead that plans needed to be put in place to operationalise the use of Flo and move from project to mainstreaming. A third business case was written for the following financial year with the objectives of further increasing usage and to put in place the processes and infrastructure to create a mainstreamed service. In order to provide the cost–benefit evidence to support this, a further evaluation which included greater numbers of patient outcomes was undertaken; it was externally reviewed by a professor from the University of Strathclyde in Scotland with an interest in TECS.

The business case was approved and requirements for mainstreaming were instigated. This began with a self-assessment using a sustainability tool[6] to check that all the necessary structure and processes were in place to ensure that a successful service was established. The action plan included the development of standard operating procedures for the service and further evaluation relating to specific disease cohorts of patients.

Operationalisation: during 2014, the requirements for operationalising TECS across Nottinghamshire were put in place. An options appraisal paper submitted to the Nottinghamshire Clinical Congress in October 2014 gave time for the recommendations to be formalised prior to the service moving from project to operational status in April 2015. This provided the Flo delivery team with clear guidance and alignment with financial and contracting activity which needed to be undertaken in line with the annual financial planning round.

The service (now known as Nottinghamshire Assistive Technology Team) continues to be hosted by Mansfield and Ashfield CCG on behalf of the rest of the health and social care community and a process for transacting costs in relation to usage of Flo was developed as a means of funding the service. Monthly reports have been set up for each organisation to identify their usage, outcomes and any issues and to highlight good practice. Regular meetings are also held with the organisation leads to discuss operational issues and provide a forum to discuss potential new usage.

Thus the programme manager is no longer required on a day-to-day basis, but is still involved locally in monthly performance meetings (which have replaced the project meetings) and Flo user events as required. The clinical lead continues to work alongside the team, offering valuable expertise and guidance, as well as providing overall confirmation and challenges.

The team continues to provide ad hoc support to other members of the large Flo 'community of practice' network (www.simple.uk.net), which also provides a great resource for identifying novel implementations of Flo and learning from others.

14. Ongoing learning and sharing good practice

The team and clinicians have co-authored a number of publications[7–12] to add to the evidence base of the deployment of TECS, share good practice and provide credibility for the local service. In addition, the team has presented at other CCGs and provider trusts. There was much interest in the joint commissioning approach, across a health and social care community, with clinical engagement and associated evaluation.

Six-monthly Flo user events continue. The emphasis has moved to clinicians and patients undertaking the presentations and setting the agendas. This also provides a good opportunity to give updates from the operational team and from the national team. Feedback is collected on what further support is required, which is fed into the next event and service development. For those who cannot attend the event, a summary newsletter is widely circulated within a week.

15. International partnerships

As part of the NHS and VA partnership scheme, Nottinghamshire hosted a visit from American colleagues with presentations by Nottinghamshire clinicians. After lunch (and a surprise visit from Robin Hood and Maid Marion!) a room full of patients and clinicians joined in to share their stories of using Flo, some of which were awe inspiring. Feedback from VA staff was that the stories were overwhelming and unforgettable.

The hosting of this event was reciprocated several months later in Washington DC, where the national clinical advocates of Flo took part in a visit which included further presentations to senior VA staff and shared learning as to how other examples of TECS (e.g. video conferencing) were in practice across the VA organisation.

16. Government interest

The team took part in a Cabinet Office 'deep dive' review of AT for long-term care which led to a government meeting to discuss evaluation and patient engagement. The programme manager, a patient and heart failure nurse met the politicians. The visit was very successful in that the MP with the national lead for TECS was satisfied that there was sufficient evidence to justify Flo as a mode of telehealth that can be used to support patients with a wide variety of health and social conditions and provide cost-effective high-quality care which results in good outcomes of care.

17. Mainstreamed service

The service became mainstreamed in April 2015, just three years after it began as a six-month 'proof of concept' project. Over 3000 patients have benefited from utilisation and the service supports over 200 staff users across 13 organisations, which includes a charity commissioned by one of the CCGs to support people with learning disabilities to live a healthier lifestyle. The success of this wide-scale initiative is also recorded in the recent publication *The Story of Parliament*.[13]

Reflections on Example 11.1

Looking back, the key to success has been having a dedicated team and service, which has enabled a continued focus on deployment of TECS, addressing perceived barriers and embedding usage into pathways.

Other examples

There are many other examples where health and social care sectors have worked together to set up pilots of TECS, such as in care homes.[14] These focus on delivery of care that supports independent living (telecare) and enhances health and well-being information exchange between patients and professionals (telehealth) and between professionals (telemedicine). Example 11.2 is one of the case studies included in this review, capturing savings made in the pilot phase.[14]

EXAMPLE 11.2   Quest for quality in care homes in Calderdale

The NHS Calderdale CCG developed a commissioning plan in 2012/13 to set up a care homes pilot that combined a multidisciplinary team, real-time access to live records for GPs, a care home matron team and telecare and telehealth systems. The aim was to encourage self-management and better care and support. The highlights two years later showed that emergency admissions were down by 25% in 2014/15, GP care home visits had reduced by 58% per annum and the cost of hospital stays had reduced by £456 000. See www.calderdaleccg.nhs.uk/tag/quest-for-quality/ and you can watch a video at www.calderdaleccg.nhs.uk/news/calderdale-care-home-initiative-in-the-running-for-a-health-service-journal-value-in-healthcare-award/

Building your own business case

Don't forget that the general public is already very technology savvy – with more than 40% of the world's population having web access, and more than 85% in the UK.[15] So you should be able to build your case on the assumption that the public will welcome the opportunity for digital delivery of their care – so long as it seems safe, convenient and meets their needs and preferences. Focus on clinical conditions or social circumstances where it is obvious (even to those who are control freaks as regards investment of funds) that there is every likelihood that a minor investment will be repaid many times over by saved healthcare usage without any or very little consequence costs; and at least as good outcomes for quality and safety of care. Long-term conditions such as asthma, COPD, diabetes and cardiovascular-related diseases are obvious foci, where it is well known that more can be done proactively at many points in the respective disease treatment pathways – by patients or clinicians. For diabetes, for instance, a recent report described one in seven hospital beds being occupied by someone with diabetes,

24 000 people with diabetes in the UK dying earlier than they need have done if they'd had best practice care and 80% of amputations being avoidable.[16]

There are examples of how to construct a business case for telehealth and which elements you should include:[17,18]

- reducing costs
- improving patient services
- avoiding hospital readmissions
- providing improved access to specialists
- educating patients
- expanding the geographic 'footprint' of the organisation (e.g. providing services across a wider area or to different groups of people).

So get a copy of the business plan template or grant application that you should complete if you are to make a successful application for funding from a particular source. Read any background information carefully to ensure that you meet the source's expectations if it is to invest in your proposed programme. Include evidence for your proposed service – look at papers published in international journals and national research and development databases (e.g. www.clahrcpp. co.uk) where you might find applications for the very long-term conditions that you wish to prioritise in the Technologies Edition of their community e-newsletter. Find reliable sources that capture cost savings if clinical teams and providers implement national guidelines for best practice clinical management, such as for proactive care of patients with chronic heart failure.[17]

BOX 11.1   Building your business case[18]

The Cisco Healthcare Business Transformation Team advises that you include:

- your operating and financial strategy (including reimbursements)
- planned deployments – based on organisational needs, desired workflow and technical requirements
- project champions: clinical (rated as most important), IT and telehealth champions
- telehealth 'architecture' or infrastructure and services, applications and devices or mobile networks, range of equipment, and connectivity
- quality standards and goals of services
- project success metrics
- training plan
- evaluation and monitoring of success.

There are practical critical factors that when collated and shared have demonstrated success in the adoption and diffusion of TECS.[12] These are:

- business requirements met
- business readiness
- training and development with strong clinical leadership
- communication of proven benefits and successes on an ongoing basis
- stakeholder engagement
- resources required over time as adoption is scaled up
- information governance and safety-giving assurance
- (clinical) governance of protocols and applications
- evaluation – of worth from range of perspectives.

While champions are critical in the early stages of a TECS programme, long-term success will only happen if the TECS are mainstreamed and owned by the organisation. Key activities must be systematised – throughout planning, launching, growing, evaluating (accepted performance metrics), commissioning, marketing and delivery stages.

References

1. www.publicservice.co.uk/news_story.asp?id=18224
2. Steventon A, Bardsley M. *The Impact of Telehealth on Use of Hospital Care and Mortality: a summary of the first findings from the Whole System Demonstrator trial.* Research Summary. London: Nuffield Trust; 2012. Available at: www.nuffieldtrust.org.uk/sites/files/nuffield/publication/120622_impact_of_telehealth_on_use_of_hospital_care_and_mortality.pdf
3. Dixon J. *Does Telehealth Reduce Hospital Costs? Six points to ponder* [blog post]. 28 June. London: Nuffield Trust; 2012. Available at: www.nuffieldtrust.org.uk/blog/does-telehealth-reduce-hospital-costs-six-points-ponder
4. www.gov.uk/government/publications/nhs-outcomes-framework-2013-to-2014
5. NHS Networks. *Welcome to AIM.* NHS Networks; n.d. Available at: www.networks.nhs.uk/nhs-networks/aim/about-us www.networks.nhs.uk/nhs-networks/aim/about-us
6. NHS Institute for Innovation and Improvement. *Sustainability: ensuring continuity in improvement.* Leeds: NHS Institute for Innovation and Improvement; 2010. Available at: www.institute.nhs.uk/sustainability_model/general/welcome_to_sustainability.html
7. Birch-Jones J. In: Chambers R *et al. Tackling Telehealth: how CCGs can commission successful telehealth services.* London: *Inside Commissioning*; 2014. p. 10. Available at: Case Study: how Nottinghamshire CCGs are tackling telehealth. http://offlinehbpl.hbpl.co.uk/NewsAttachments/GCC/Inside_Commissioning_Tackling_Telehealth.pdf
8. Birch-Jones J. In: Chambers R *et al. Tackling Telehealth: how CCGs can commission successful telehealth services.* London: *Inside Commissioning*; 2014. Available at: http://offlinehbpl.hbpl.co.uk/NewsAttachments/GCC/Inside_Commissioning_Tackling_Telehealth.pdf
9. Birch-Jones J. In: Chambers R *et al. Tackling Telehealth: how CCGs can commission successful telehealth services.* London: *Inside Commissioning*; 2014. Available at: http://offlinehbpl.hbpl.co.uk/NewsAttachments/GCC/Inside_Commissioning_Tackling_Telehealth.pdf

10. Cund A, Birch-Jones J, Kay M *et al*. Self-management: keeping it simple with Flo. *Nursing (Auckl)*. 2015; **5**: 49–55.

11. Holmes M, Clark S. Technology-enabled care services: novel method of managing liver disease. *Gastrointest Nurs (Liver Nurs Suppl)* 2014; **12**(Suppl. 10): S22–7. doi: 10.12968/gasn.2014.12.Sup10.S22

12. Taylor L, Birch-Jones J. Implementing a technology enabled care service. *Br J Healthc Manag*. 2016; **22**(1): 224–34.

13. History of Parliament Trust. *The Story of Parliament: celebrating 750 years of parliament in Britain*. London: Regal Press; 2015. Available at: http://content.yudu.com/web/3f4fn/0A3pn76/TheStoryofParliament/flash/resources/index.htm?referrerUrl

14. NHS England. *Quick Guide: technology in care homes; transforming urgent and emergency care services in England*. Leeds: NHS England; n.d. Available at: www.nhs.uk/NHSEngland/keogh-review/Documents/quick-guides/quick-guide-technology-in-care-homes.pdf

15. Ofcom. *Internet Use and Attitudes: 2015 metrics bulletin*. London: Ofcom; 2015. Available at: http://stakeholders.ofcom.org.uk/binaries/research/cmr/cmr15/Internet_use_and_attitudes_bulletin.pdf

16. Diabetes UK. *The Cost of Diabetes: report*. London: Diabetes UK; 2014. Available at: www.diabetes.org.uk

17. Alderwick H, Robertson R, Appleby J *et al*. *Better Value in the NHS: the role of changes in clinical practice*. London: The King's Fund; 2015. Available at: www.kingsfund.org.uk/sites/files/kf/field/field_publication_file/better-value-nhs-Kings-Fund-July%202015.pdf

18. Mortensen J. *Cisco Approach to Telehealth: a viewpoint from the Cisco Healthcare Business Transformation Team*. San Jose, CA: Cisco; 2015. Available at: www.cisco.com/web/strategy/docs/healthcare/cisco-approach-to-telehealth.pdf

Chapter 12

Managing risks of technology enabled care services

Jayne Birch-Jones, Dr Ruth Chambers

You do need to anticipate and manage risks associated with implementing technology enabled care services (TECS) to be effective. This includes data sharing, informed patient consent, device management and other information governance and clinical safety issues. Risk management is an essential component of clinical governance too.

Risk assessment

Risk is the probability that a hazard will give rise to harm. But the extent to which you judge that a harmful outcome is likely to occur and that likely outcome is to be harmful is subjective. So you need to set up systems that minimise the likelihood of harm happening from public or patient, care professional or manager and organisational perspectives. On the whole, people tend to be over-optimistic about risk occurring so there is a high probability that risk(s) will be underestimated.[1]

Risk management at an organisational level (trust, Clinical Commissioning Group [CCG] or practice) mainly centres on 'facts' rather than 'values' or 'preferences'. This is the probability that a hazard will give rise to harm – how bad is that risk, how likely is it, when might the risk happen (if ever) and how certain are leaders of their estimates about the risks? This applies just as much whether the risk is an environmental or organisational risk in the organisation, or a clinical risk.

Risk assessment establishes actual levels of risk. It should lead to action to prevent or control those risks to people or the organisation or business that otherwise might be affected. Risk assessment entails the scientific assessment of the size and nature of a risk which is followed by a decision on whether to:

- transfer the risk
- negate the risk
- share the risk
- ignore the risk
- accept the risk.

Risk management

The type of action or inaction you opt for will depend on the probability of the risk occurring or recurring, the impact of the risk if it should happen and the costs of preventing or avoiding the risk(s).

The four stages in risk management[2] are to:

- identify key risks and any triggers, encouraging staff to volunteer and discuss observed risks and adverse events
- analyse the risk – how common is it, are there patterns or trends, what impact does it have, does that impact matter, how frequent might high-risk occurrences be?
- control the risk – what you can do about it, implement changes in practice as necessary, feedback to staff
- cost the risk – look at the cost of getting it right versus the cost of a risky outcome.

Risks occur whether or not you introduce a new intervention or patient pathway such as TECS. There may be risks that people forget or ignore as the new system or procedure is introduced, or they are unaware of when communication is poor or non-existent. But you do need to introduce new interventions or ways of doing things such as TECS, otherwise you will be in danger of perpetuating outdated practices or not being sufficiently flexible to meet new or rising demands.

Sometimes there are consequence costs which also need to be envisaged and minimised. Managing or controlling one risk may have a knock-on effect of creating new or greater risks elsewhere. If you do not have a grasp of the bigger picture, you can make things worse – and more risky.

Risk management when implementing TECS

Managing and communicating risk is integral to clinical governance, whether at an individual patient level or at an organisational level. Clinical governance is about doing anything and everything required to maximise the quality of delivery of care and clinical effectiveness. Risk management is central to a strong clinical governance culture where quality is considered in as wide a perspective as possible to:

- sustain quality improvements over time
- minimise inequalities in the health of different sub-groups of the population
- reduce variations in the provision of healthcare services
- define standards.

Clinical risk management will focus on identifying and prioritising individuals most at risk of adverse effects of ill-health if their condition is not treated effectively or managed well over the long term; organisational risk management will ensure that the systems and procedures necessary to achieve excellent clinical management are in place all of the time. TECS risk management is integral to this culture. This might be by:

- individualising the treatment and management plan of a patient or service user according to their values, personal preferences and beliefs; explaining the risks and benefits of various TECS options to give them an informed choice
- targeting TECS in such a way as to include those at most risk of the condition – including attention to their health or social care setting, timing, surroundings and reminders
- basing all TECS on the best evidence, and where that is not available evaluating care and treatment or linking to larger studies that aim to provide evidence
- making sure that all care professionals are clear about their roles and responsibilities, especially where treatment or TECS set-up is started by one professional and monitored at intervals, while other health professionals provide interim everyday care
- reducing waiting times for TECS – prioritising people's care in line with a clinical care pathway or other agreed protocol. Ensuring that there are no time delays when patients pass from one specialist or setting to another
- managing resources and services to ration and prioritise care such that those with the most needs receive appropriate treatment and investigations as soon as possible.

Completing information governance requirements

When implementing TECS, health or social care, organisations should be aware of national information governance (IG) considerations and also follow their own internal IG and clinical safety policies and procedures.

Depending on the type of TECS being implemented, the following should be considered:

- *Information Governance Toolkit* compliance[3]
- clinical risk management standards, e.g. ISB 0160,[4] ISO[5]
- *The Interoperability Toolkit*[6]
- Medicines and Healthcare Regulatory Agency (MHRA) *Medical Devices Regulation and Safety*[7]
- MHRA *Medical Devices: software applications (apps)*[8]
- Telecare Services Association (TSA) *Integrated Code of Practice*[9]
- *Telecare Services Code of Practice for Europe.*[10]

Organisational IG teams should be involved in the early stages of TECS implementation planning to ensure that they have input into evaluating the product and highlighting and providing guidance on any potential IG issues.

Data sharing

National and local data sharing policies and procedures should be adhered to when considering the implementation of TECS, in particular the identification of a lead with responsibility for the ongoing fair processing campaign to inform patients about the use of their data. Data sharing considerations should cover:

- processes and legislation (including the completion of a privacy impact assessment)
- people (training and education)
- technology being used.

Privacy Impact Assessment (PIA)

You would complete a PIA to assess privacy risks in the collection, use and disclosure of personal information. You should identify and mitigate any data protection and privacy concerns at the initiation of a project so that any personal and sensitive information requirements are complied with. Include data protection compliance from the start rather than try to bolt it on once you have the project up and running.

A PIA should be completed whenever there is a change in your delivery of TECS that is likely to involve a new or revised way in which personal data is handled such as with a redesign of a process or service (e.g. set up Skype for clinical consultations); a new process or electronic information source is set up that collects and holds personal data; or your organisation plans to use, monitor or report personal information in different ways. Undertaking evaluation might mean a change to data sharing agreements. (For more information see www.ico.org.uk)

Informed patient consent

Consent to treatment is a voluntary and continuing permission by the patient to receive a particular treatment (or in this case mode of treatment or intervention) based on an adequate knowledge of the purpose, nature and likely risks, including the likelihood of success and any alternatives to that treatment or mode of consultation. Consent can be verbal, written or implied; implied consent is compliance by a patient with a particular treatment, examination or mode of consultation in a non-verbal way.

IG colleagues will advise on ensuring that the most appropriate processes and documentation for patient consent are met. Gaining patient consent also needs to be part of staff training and written into TECS standard operating procedures. Written consent from the patient or their legal representative must be gained prior to the first remote consultation and will be confirmed verbally prior to any following remote consultations. In accordance with the Mental Capacity Act 2005,[11] there is a presumption of capacity until proven otherwise. If a patient is deemed to lack capacity for a decision at a given time, despite efforts to assist them in understanding the nature of the decision that is to be made, a personal representative who has lasting power of attorney for their health and welfare can do this on their behalf.

Devices

When considering the procurement of TECS-related devices, input from colleagues with expertise in medical equipment should be involved to advise on medical device certification and safety checks, such as portable appliance testing (PAT). In addition an evaluation of data integrity, data accuracy, IT standards, regulation and governance adherence needs to be undertaken. Data validation and data quality processes need to be followed as part of implementation.

EXAMPLE 12.1 TECS clinical safety process

Nottinghamshire local health and social care community mainstreamed the use of a TECS system in April 2015. As part of this process, a clinical safety assessment was undertaken in line with the Health and Social Care Information Centre (HSCIC) ISB 0160: clinical risk management – its application in the deployment and use of health IT systems.[12]

The evidence to support the assessment included a:

- hazard log
- risks and issues log
- quality impact assessment
- privacy impact assessment.

Scrutinising this document (*see* Appendix 1) will give you insights into the scope and depth of such a risk assessment for your organisation. This relays the associated reviewed patient safety closure report and Clinical Authority to Deploy (CATD) for the Flo simple telehealth system, as signed off by the CCG's clinical safety officer. This review process might be adapted or amended for any mode of delivery of TECS.

FAQs

Q1. How can you interact or involve the public or individuals in decision making about risks and benefits of TECS?

A. There is a variety of qualitative methods used to gather information and views from patients, carers and the general public, such as:

- focus groups and discussion groups
- special interest patient groups: user groups, carer groups, patient participation groups, disease support groups
- general public opinion: opinion polls, citizens juries, standing panels, public meetings, neighbourhood forums
- community development: local community development projects, healthy living centre activities
- consensus events or activities: Delphi surveys, nominal groups, consensus development conferences
- informal feedback from patients: in-house systems such as suggestion boxes and complaints.

Use a variety of consultation methods which include options to give information, receive information, allow interchange of views between professionals and the public – and allow opportunities for the public to reflect before formulating their views after hearing the opinions of experts or other members of the public.

Q2. How can we reduce the risks of disjointed care as patients cross from one setting to another if there is no agreement about the evidence for best practice or use of TECS across these interfaces?

A. There are many historical blocks and barriers to team working and partnership working across NHS settings or between health and social care organisations. Risk management will involve:

- devising clinical care pathways as an agreed timed framework for treating the most common conditions; this will increase the 'seamlessness' of care across the primary-secondary-community care interfaces
- encouraging ownership of clinical care pathways by involving

representatives of all professional and managerial interests in devising and reviewing the pathways

- thinking as widely as possible about a health condition so that all organisations with an influence on the outcome of that particular condition contribute to drawing up and applying that pathway; for instance, a TECS pathway for people suffering from dementia will involve social workers, financial advisers, housing officers, voluntary groups and others as well as clinicians and managers working in the NHS.

References

1. Mohanna K, Chambers R. *Risk Matters in Healthcare: communicating, explaining and managing risk.* Abingdon: Radcliffe Medical Press; 2000.
2. Lilley R, Lambden P. *Making Sense of Risk Management: a workbook for primary care.* Oxford: Radcliffe Medical Press; 1999.
3. Health and Social Care Information Centre (HSCIC). *Information Governance Toolkit.* Leeds: HSCIC; 2015. Available at: www.igt.hscic.gov.uk/
4. HSCIC. ISB 0160 Clinical Risk Management: its application in the deployment and use of health IT systems. In: *Clinical Risk Management Standards.* Leeds: HSCIC; 2015. Available at: http://systems.hscic.gov.uk/clinsafety/dscn
5. ISO/TS 13131:2014. Health Informatics: telehealth services – quality planning guidelines. Geneva: International Organization for Standardization (ISO); 2014. Available at: www.iso.org/iso/iso_catalogue/catalogue_tc/catalogue_detail.htm?csnumber=53052
6. HSCIC. *The Interoperability Toolkit.* Leeds: HSCIC; 2015. Available at: http://systems.hscic.gov.uk/interop/itk
7. Medicines and Healthcare Products Regulatory Agency (MHRA), Department of Health. *Medical Devices Regulation and Safety.* London: MHRA; 2015. Available at: www.gov.uk/topic/medicines-medical-devices-blood/medical-devices-regulation-safety
8. MHRA. *Medical Devices: software applications (apps).* London: MHRA; 2015. Available at: www.gov.uk/government/publications/medical-devices-software-applications-apps
9. Telecare Service Association (TSA). *Integrated Code of Practice.* Wilmslow: TSA; n.d. Available at: www.telecare.org.uk/standards/telecare-code-of-practice
10. TeleSCoPE Project. *Telehealth Services Code of Practice for Europe.* TeleSCoPE Project; 2015. Available at: www.telehealthcode.eu/
11. Mental Capacity Act 2005. Available at: www.gov.uk/government/collections/mental-capacity-act-making-decisions
12. Compliance assessment. In: ISB 0160: clinical risk management – its application in the deployment and use of health IT systems. Version 2. Leeds: HSCIC; 2013. Available at: www.hscic.gov.uk/media/17259/0160compliancev2/xls/0160compliancev2.xlsx

NHS

Mansfield and Ashfield
Clinical Commissioning Group

Appendix 1: Example of reviewed patient safety closure report and clinical authority to deploy (CATD) for Flo simple telehealth (STH) by one CCG

Document location:
The current master version of this document is stored:

Document author:

Author	Role	Signature

Document amendment history:

Document version	Date amended	Amended by	Brief summary of changes

Formal approval:

Name	Signature	Title/Responsibility	Date	Version

Distribution:

1. Introduction

In a much overdue response to concerns about patient safety in the design of IT software, NHS trusts are mandated by Data Set Change Notice (DSCN) 18/2009 (updated to ISB 0160 v3.1 issued 28 May 2013) to be able to demonstrate that robust processes are in place to check the software that is procured by trusts (and also existing clinical systems) is appropriately assessed from a 'patient safety' perspective. This document is a component part of the processes that have been put in place in order to adhere to patient safety requirements and formally evidences that these processes have taken place.

The system has been deployed in a limited fashion locally (although more extensively in other parts of the NHS), but this deployment continues the process and mainstreams the system, adhering to the revised ISO 0160 v3.1

documentation released by HSCIC in May 2013. This documentation covers essentially the same points as the original but gives further clarity.

2. Background

In England 15.4 million people in England (2013 figures) have a long-term condition (LTC). The UK has an ageing population, and with the prevalence rates of LTCs increasing sharply to over 60% in patients over 60 years, the percentage of people with LTCs looks set to increase. LTC patients use disproportionately more primary and secondary care services – 52% of GP appointments, 65% of all outpatient appointments, and 72% of all inpatient bed days.

Evidence suggests that telehealth allows patients to set and achieve goals around self-care, increasing proactive personal management of their conditions, and improving health outcomes. The readmission rates for chronic obstructive pulmonary disease (COPD) are >20% against an overall readmission average of 6.7%.

The aim of the project was to deploy Flo across the local health community where clinicians prioritise a need, and over 1200 patients have now utilised Flo locally with no untoward incidents.

3. Intended use

- Regularly collect, monitor and alert on any biometric observation or question tree and many validated questionnaires.
- Improve concordance with treatment regimens through encouragement, reminders and interactive contact.
- Enable improvements in clinical team productivity and outcome quality.
- Engage patients in their health and social care pathways and services.
- Due to the ultra-low cost of STH, its ease of use and universal acceptability of the methods, STH is affordable and deployable on an unequalled scale across an unrivalled range of conditions and pathways.

Productivity gains

- Increase in community matrons or nurse caseloads
- GP reduction in home visits or surgery appointments
- Reduced hospital admission rates

Patient benefits

- Increase in patients' quality of life
- Reduced costs or travelling time for patients
- Reduced time off work

These quantitative and qualitative indicators will be measured and realised as part of the project. Section 4 provides indicative direct, secondary and net benefits.

Flo introduces the following functionality.

- The ability to receive biometric readings from a patient via SMS text messaging from any mobile phone and operator.
- The ability to monitor and set alerts based on individual patient parameters that informs the patient what to do, therefore promoting self-care, and supports the clinician's ability to triage and increase monitoring without the need for additional visits or clinic appointments.

Clinicians will assess patient suitability on a visit, utilise the Patient Recruitment Pack and gain consent. Exclusions may exist whereby a patient cannot use a mobile phone, although future developments may include the use of landlines. When a patient consents to using Flo the opt in message and response from the patient will not only test the patient's ability to respond but also the signal coverage in their area.

4. *Clinical hazards and mitigation*

A Patient Safety Hazard Group has been set up through utilising the clinicians currently involved in using Flo and their patients.

There are seven hazards that have been identified. All have mitigations and have been accepted to be tolerated. The Hazard Patient Safety Testing Group comprises of the project team members and the clinicians already deploying Flo in Nottinghamshire.

The hazard analysis has been reviewed with no additional hazards identified and the documentation can be located:……..

A formal review and assessment for the ISB 0160 has been conducted and the following table summarises the compliance of Flo Simple Telehealth:

Section	Heading	Levels of Compliance					
		Yes	No	Not Applicable	Awaiting	Partial	Outstanding
2	General requirements	12	0	2	1*	0	0
3	Project safety documentation and repositories	23	0	0	0	0	0
4	Clinical risk analysis	9	0	0	0	0	0
5	Clinical risk evaluation	4	0	0	0	0	0
6	Clinical risk control	13	0	0	0	0	0
7	Deployment, maintenance and decommissioning	12	0	7	0	0	0
	Total	73	0	9	1	0	0

Area	Level of Compliance					
	Yes	No	Not applicable	Awaiting	Partial	Outstanding
Management system	15	0	2	0	0	0
Project	58	0	7	1	0	0
Total	73	0	9	1	0	0

* The entry under Section 2 – General requirements in the awaiting column is due to the absence of a supplier safety case

Any new release from the Flo system is circulated to all clinicians using the system. The changes are also tested by the assistive technology (AT) team to ensure that there are no adverse effects or patient safety issues. Training is also provided and circulated to all clinical users of Flo.

5. Conclusion

An evaluation report has been published and circulated to all CCGs highlighting patient and clinician response and outcomes; this can be shared upon request. There have also been a number of publications, one of which was a randomised control trial which is available upon request.

- Flo has been sufficiently tested to assure its safety through its use led by NHS Stoke-on-Trent with 23 000 patients using 120 different protocols nationally; locally over 1200 patients have utilised the system.
- Mediaburst has undertaken the IG toolkit. Compliance with requirement 4.3.1 of ISB 0129 version 2 is not evidenced. However, an additional check of our operating procedures and testing approach added an additional level of assurance. Also the intended use of Flo is decided and controlled at a local level.
- Each organisation adopting Flo follows its own risk management processes and any protocol written is approved clinically with clinical authority to deploy approval required. Flo and some national protocols have national coverage or sign-off but under local processes; for ease of working the adoption processes and procedures are shared and local testing is still undertaken.
- Clinical authority to deploy as a mainstreamed service is being sought for the Flo deployment with annual reviews as part of services provision and KPIs [Key Performance Indicators].

All quantitative and qualitative data analysis will be made available as part of an annual review across the local health community. Each deployment will be planned using Prince2 Project management and any issues or risks highlighted and reported to the work stream. It is emphasised during patient sign-up that this is not an emergency service and therefore does not replace any current access to services.

Although the supplier has not presented a safety case in compliance with ISB 0129 I am satisfied that the requirements are covered within this safety case for the deployment, as the risks have been appropriately tested locally and the larger deployments of the same system within the NHS have not shown any other risks.

There are appropriate security procedures in place to prevent the release or corruption of the data by unauthorised persons and data remains completely within the UK.

There is an appropriate data retention policy and when a patient ceases to be involved with the programme their clinical data is transferred to their clinical digital record, e.g. SystmOne, by the clinician prior to deletion of the record.

The initial hazard log has been updated in the light of experience with the initial deployment and this deployment.

The system does not change or advise on clinical care. It merely brings biometric measurements to the attention of the supervising clinician in a controlled manner to enhance timely decision making.

Excellent local processes exist to identify and report any risks which emerge. They also give good training and business management systems which will allow a controlled safe deployment.

There are no deviations from accepted practices which would jeopardise a safe deployment.

I am satisfied that the product is clinically safe to continue to deploy without limitation, according to the project plan.

(Signature)
Clinical Safety Officer

Chapter 13

Overcoming resistance and maximising opportunities for the adoption of technology enabled care services

Lisa Taylor

Introduction

Digital healthcare is developing at an exponential rate and has quickly harvested the interest of global technology and pharmaceutical companies; yet there is a wide variability across Europe and beyond in its maturity.[1] Despite the many drivers to adopt new models of care and innovation in the NHS,[2] adoption and diffusion of technology enabled care services (TECS) is still very variable in relation to its existence and impact. Those working in health and social care need to overcome the characteristic challenges for their organisation, clinicians and patients or service users to enable the necessary diffusion, if TECS is to be an integral part of how today's healthcare is delivered.

We must recognise the differing contexts for influencing new clinical practice that organisations provide as well as focusing on the importance of organisational strategy and implementation planning for delivery of TECS and associated service developments in generating cost savings alongside improved patient satisfaction and clinical outcomes. Building on existing cultural and structural features will significantly influence the likelihood that TECS will be successfully embedded as routine care.

Cultural impact

System readiness for innovation,[3] whereby an organisation appears amenable to the concept of innovation but not ready or willing to create an environment conducive to its success, remains a strong determining factor of the speed at which TECS is embraced as a viable option for care delivery in health or social care settings. An organisation should nurture a culture amenable to the use of technology, thereby granting *'permission'* for colleagues to make best use of TECS. The presence or absence of a culture that stimulates, or provides permission for, TECS within its care or service delivery mechanisms will dictate the likelihood of success, regardless of its own quality or potential. The identification of organisation-wide clinical and managerial leadership accelerates the stimulation of awareness and positioning of TECS. Enriching clinician–managerial relationships also enhances communication and identification of common ground when seeking to adopt or further develop use of TECS.

The stakeholders involved in delivery of TECS is another complex matter, varying between services and health economies and changes over time with emerging confusion over required consultation, involvement and leadership. In early adoption it is useful to consult widely but distil key leaders to form an effective stakeholder group so as not to create an overly complex structure.

Organisations will always demonstrate their own tensions for change[3] – a characteristic dictating the speed at which healthcare delivery changes from where it is today, to where it needs to be to meet ever-increasing demands. The presence, communication and clinical acknowledgement of organisational drivers for change improve the willingness with which innovative practice is considered, stretching the organisation's tension for change. The fit between delivery of TECS and current organisational values and strategic aims, combined with a clear understanding among clinical teams of how the integration of TECS fits with the organisational vision, further supports successful adoption.

An organisation with a supportive, enthusiastic culture that permits open discussion around current practice that is not risk averse and champions the testing of new ideas is an excellent starting point for the introduction of TECS. Where cross-boundary working is encouraged and supportive human resources strategies exist, then permission to change is provided by default, creating an environment where TECS can thrive. Organisational culture is highly influential in determining the likelihood of the integration of TECS as modes of delivery of usual care. Several cultural assessment tools, such as those from The King's Fund,[4] are available and offer an opportunity to understand the current situation in your organisation and highlight areas for improvement and development.

Equipping the workforce

Working to create a supportive environment within your organisation and the wider health economy further enhances the potential for scalability and exploiting opportunities for cross-boundary collaborations for TECS. Effective engagement with others across health and social care is key. Impact and the chance of sustainability escalate significantly where TECS underpins integrated care coordinated along patient pathways between the NHS, social care and other local provider organisations. Developing or enhancing information and clinical governance policies reduces any perceived individual risks of changing clinical practice and improves confidence in working differently.

Utilising existing best practice in the implementation and delivery of TECS through cross-boundary working also provides reassurance, further promoting a culture amenable to innovation. Speed of adoption of pathways is increased with the development of organisational forums aimed at sharing learning, thus exposing new and potential TECS adopters to a pool of existing knowledge.

Making best use of current national resources also prepares and educates an organisation for the integration of TECS in the provision of care. A national TECS online resource for commissioners has been developed to help maximise the value of TECS across the whole health economy.[5] This and other such resources raise awareness of a wide range of benefits of TECS, for information on how to commission, procure, implement and evaluate these types of solutions effectively.

Both clinical users and patients or service users should feel that technology supports them better and is not an added burden to their already busy schedules. If clinical users do not feel supported to change and use different modes of TECS, adoption will never happen, be slow or cease to exist. Therefore strategies to provide ongoing support and training for both patients and staff are essential. Dedicated time to implement TECS along with the capacity to evaluate its impact is vital in creating an environment for innovation to thrive.[3] Where organisations commit to supporting changes in working practices by recognising education and training as a key determinant of success for delivery,[6] adoption of TECS proves easier. The development of clear basic competences as part of organisational mandatory training would ensure that staff are supported as well as providing a clear signal that technology is accepted standard practice across the organisation. Supporting the necessary changes in workforce and role redesign to equip the current and future workforce in fully exploiting the development of TECS breeds confidence and increases the perception that TECS are an accepted mode of care.

EXAMPLE 13.1   Clinician's continued professional development (CPD) programme for digital healthcare[7]

Stoke-on-Trent Clinical Commissioning Group (CCG) has developed an online CPD programme to support the development of a supportive workplace culture within which to deploy remote technology to support, encourage, monitor and manage patients or service users. The course is available for both clinicians and managers and includes practical tools aimed at enabling teams to use learning and development activities to improve their experience with modes of digital delivery of care.[7] The course has been developed to support learning about connected health in general yet with a specific focus on Florence simple telehealth. The CPD programme encourages the participant to put their learning into practice.

Nationally, support to incorporate core competences for delivery of TECS into workforce development is emerging. But when teams are just starting out with TECS, it is important to appoint the best-placed or appropriately skilled member of the team to lead implementation, with access to willing wider support as needed. TECS champions and local enthusiasts can engage, train and drive forward improvements. But to sustain momentum a formalised role is more effective long term. Organisations may wish to access external support and training where available to develop TECS capabilities within the current skill mix to assist early planning, increasing the rate and success of adoption and ultimate sustainability. They might also enable connections with existing internal and external adopters of TECS to access current knowledge. This develops the organisation's absorptive capacity[8] and also offers opportunities in identifying the true value of TECS; where such collaboration is lacking an organisation's absorptive capacity is reduced and an incompatible environment for innovation emerges.[9]

Maximising effective clinical champions

Often the limiting factor in effective deployment of a new service is incomplete buy-in from staff or patients rather than any limitation in the supportive

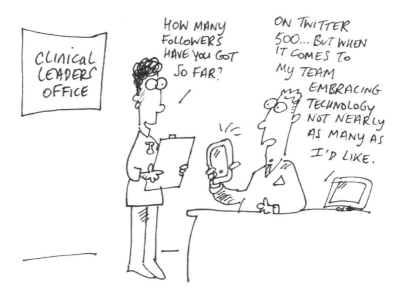

technology or redesigned pathway. Clinical oversight, acceptance and championing of TECS as a feasible model of care is essential for their development and ultimate sustainability and should be considered as a key determinant of success. Harnessing effective clinical leadership to actively champion TECS at an organisational level ensures clinical relevance and opportunities for exploitation of strategic and operational opportunities across the organisation. Where clinical leadership has been weak or not prioritised, adoption and subsequent mainstreaming prove more challenging.

The role of clinical leader for TECS

Successful clinical leads in TECS actively inspire and motivate their colleagues, helping to distil intelligence around integration of TECS. The clinical leader seeks opportunities to identify areas for the introduction of TECS in line with local disease prevalence and clinical and business priorities, while recognising the organisation's overall transformation plans, ensuring that provision of TECS is aligned to clinical service delivery requirements. The clinical leader also has the opportunity to use existing channels to exploit opportunities for effective communication with regard to opportunities and outcomes of TECS use across the organisation and beyond. Governance is also assured around new TECS applications, ensuring alignment with current best practice and clinical guidelines where available, not only assuring patient safety but also instilling confidence with clinical colleagues over their adoption.

Clinical engagement is also essential in ensuring that TECS incorporate both health or social care professional and patient or service user need in its design and that clinicians feel 'in control of how they shape services, with local innovation not stifled by heavy national overlay'.[6] The engagement of regional clinical networks with the expertise of viewing pathways across organisational boundaries when developing demand and stimulus for TECS supplements clinical oversight and enhances confidence; yet care should be taken that such interaction does not delay or confuse local priorities. Local clinical and organisational ownership can minimise any disruption to workflow caused by the introduction of TECS and opportunities for the visibility of associated benefits. Assurance around accurate communication of the purpose of TECS and intention is also generated. This eases commonly held fears that new ways of working increase workload or may be paving the way for a reduced headcount.

Organisational strategies should harness the influence of known local clinical opinion leaders, particularly early in the development of TECS, so increasing the likelihood of success. Where this is lacking, adoption is delayed or diffusion may be limited. Additional identification and engagement of internal 'clinical champions' to lead adoption through to sustainability for TECS help the wider team and strengthens cross-boundary and network relationships.

To emerge as clinical champions, clinicians must be exposed to enough good-quality information to be clear about the 'relative advantages' that TECS hold over and above current practice and be willing to communicate widely so that colleagues change their current behaviour and practice.[3] Any proposed TECS model must clearly demonstrate how it will bring added value to the current process, pathway or system.[10] The notion of added value is based on the accepted reality that not all change is positive and deserving of reproduction. In the current climate of extensive change, it is perhaps demonstrating the added value or relative advantage of a particular TECS model that enables it to justify investment against the backdrop of other potentially deserving ideas – proven or otherwise. Such added value and relative advantage should contain clear demonstrable qualities, whether these are clinical, financial or quality, that are highly rated by all stakeholders, further enhancing the 'value proposition'.[10] Demonstration of these qualities will influence organisational decisions to adopt, or their motivation to sustain TECS.[3] They should ideally be demonstrated by existing evidence or by sharing best practice.[6]

Active clinical and managerial champions are key determinants to the embedment of TECS; however, with the recent reorganisation in health and social care across all sectors, roles have often been lost or refocused. Consistency of both clinical and managerial TECS leads enhances the speed of integration while securing an organisational memory as a platform for further expansion and sustainability of TECS.

Navigating the options

Such fast development, availability and scope of different healthcare technology can be overwhelming for clinician and patient or service user, making the appreciation of its relative advantages even more bewildering. Therefore it is paramount that any chosen technology supports an existing clinical or efficiency need, and not vice versa. The chosen model must be relevant to tasks planned or undertaken, not overly complex and be able to be trialled on a limited basis to encourage implementation,[3] while also improving clinical outcomes and assessing its impact.

One of the most-cited concerns expressed by clinicians is the lack of availability of good-quality outcome data, including cost savings and benefits expected from TECS. The evidence base for using technology to enhance care is large, complex and continuing to grow rapidly. TECS are complex interventions involving people, processes and technology and any derived outcomes have dependencies across all of these elements. Currently available evidence is based on a wide range of TECS methodologies and subsequently provides varied messages on clinical versus cost-effective outcomes, such as the various published contradictory findings around the cost-effectiveness of the 2010 Whole System Demonstrator remote monitoring telehealth pilot.[11]

Inconclusive findings from any implementation of TECS can create an opportunity for those already hesitant to cite lack of evidence as mitigation for refusal to support adoption of TECS as a whole. Although such reports relay only a small part of the TECS story they can generate negative opinion about TECS integration in general. The rapid progress in the market in recent years has seen both the breadth and intelligence around TECS widen. This has brought about more effective solutions being deployed quicker and at less cost and goes some way to reducing the impact of such inconclusive outcomes. However, the importance of being able to access good-quality, clear information in improving awareness of today's deployment of TECS cannot be underestimated. This makes it easier for potential adopters to digest the distinction between the varieties of TECS models with clear, evidenced messages around their own relative advantages over normal care.

EXAMPLE 13.2 Simple telehealth collaborative community facilitating adoption

Flo simple telehealth was introduced in 2010 as an NHS designed and owned self-management tool supporting patients to engage with their own health and adhere better to therapies and shared care management plans. Patients are helped to help themselves to improve adherence and gain confidence with their existing pathway or treatment though a mix of automated and interactive communications.[12]

One of the main enablers of Flo's successful adoption across the UK has been the establishment and growth of its own collaborative community developed to enable communication around the proven value and benefits of Flo's integration between peers. Enabling peer-to-peer networking has demonstrated a variety of advantages in promoting Flo's growth. The collaborative community harnessed the learning of early adopters and played an important role in growing clinical confidence, and remains doing so for new and emerging pathways. Primarily, due to the innovative nature of Flo both as a product and also in the scope of its application, the collaborative community provides a trusted environment for those new to adoption to gain an honest appraisal of its value, providing credibility and confidence over its use. The collaborative community also enables successful locally developed applications to spread beyond their original boundary, providing a more efficient approach to dissemination, and ultimately a richer evidence base. Organisations within the collaborative community also find it useful to develop their own local peer-to-peer sharing networks to secure organisational awareness, knowledge and retention of best practice.

One useful approach is to enable new and existing users of TECS to interact. This helps build credibility and confidence over the proposed use while enabling peer-to-peer understanding around its breadth and effectiveness. NHS England is commited[13] to developing a number of 'test-bed' sites aimed at deploying and evaluating the impact of different technologies and innovations; this should enhance the potential for increased availability of evidence-based practice.

Sharing available focused evidence such as from the national TECS evidence base[14] facilitates access to a variety of outcomes and enhances opportunities for informed choices to match local need and technological fit. Challenges remain over further availability and inclusiveness of evidence given the pace and scope of the market for TECS.

At an organisational level, evaluating local usage of TECS is essential. Sharing widely not only the benefits realised but also areas for improvement enables teams to learn in their expansion phase and increases the likelihood of the sustainability and diffusion of TECS. Where this is lacking, motivation to sustain implementation can dwindle.

The benefits of any new advances in health or social care delivery, such as TECS, are being quickly incorporated into the delivery of nationally recommended practice, such as the introduction of NICE guidelines to provide synergy, improve confidence and the likelihood of clinicians adopting TECS. Therefore it is sensible to align the deployment of TECS with current clinical guidelines or best practice, or where current guidance is lacking using technology to enhance the delivery of such accepted pathways.

Enhancing patient or service user acceptance

The power held by the patient or service user in both accepting and championing TECS is essential to its growth. Understanding the factors that influence patients taking up and continuing to access TECS is therefore fundamental to its sustainability.[15] However, not all patients will be suitable for TECS as dictated by their condition, suitability or choice. Acknowledging that TECS may not provide the best fit for each and every patient or service user is essential in targeting resources efficiently and maintaining clinical energy. Ensuring that patients who are being offered TECS understand why they are being asked to use it and the benefits it offers enhances patient acceptance and ultimately helps to secure their engagement.

A preference, perceived or otherwise, for face-to-face care can be one of the main barriers to patient acceptance of telehealth.[15] Informed discussions with patients around the purpose, benefits and added value of TECS combined with clinicians having the flexibility to titrate the introduction of technology more slowly and at the right time should help. Many patients appreciate their current face-to-face healthcare. So take the opportunity to explain that with the introduction of TECS, such interactions and oversight may increase, albeit in different ways.

Culture also impacts heavily on a patient's acceptance of TECS as a viable alternative to the models of care they have either commonly experienced or have come to expect. Provision of TECS *is* a new model of care and challenges the culture of how healthcare is delivered; so in the same way that NHS professionals benefit from education regarding their worth, so do patients or service users. By increasing and championing awareness of TECS to patients, their confidence and ultimately acceptance levels will increase. Using existing communication channels to champion real patient stories around their use of TECS, including notice boards, newsletters, local press or videos, are all effective methods to increase public awareness.

Harnessing the voice of local patient groups also provides an environment for much needed consultation and engagement. Listening to colleagues and patients both as potential and new users is essential and provides valuable insights to help shape future TECS delivery.

From a patient's perspective, the provision of TECS reinforced by clinicians who are confident about their purpose and mode of delivery goes a long way to transmitting confidence that technology enabled care is an accepted, safe model of care. Once introduced to TECS, patient or service user confidence is also sustained by having access to patient-focused, good-quality, reliable equipment that causes minimal disruption to their healthcare or everyday life. Access to such technology also minimises staff workload.

FAQs

Q1 Are there any particular measures of perception and patient satisfaction you'd recommend?

A. Capturing patient perception and satisfaction around their use of TECS is essential to inform new pathways, distil successes and learn from the challenges experienced both during and after their use. Validated measures include a telehealth acceptance questionnaire[16] developed by the Universities of Sheffield and Manchester to assess motivation in a patient's use of telehealth; this was aimed at identifying those patients who were likely to abandon telehealth.[15] However, local evaluation matched to existing purpose of use might also generate feedback to add quality and intelligence. Such feedback is invaluable to ensure that any integration of TECS in usual care is delivering on its intentions, to inform any necessary improvements and ultimately to increase the likelihood of TECS being mainstreamed.

Q2 What are your top tips on overcoming barriers to the adoption of TECS?

A. To overcome barriers to TECS and maximise adoption, you need to secure the hearts and minds of potential adopters and enablers. Interaction between such advocates provides a cumulative effect. This challenge extends not only to clinical and social care colleagues but also to organisational leadership and most certainly patients and potential service users if there is to be wide acceptance of technology playing an integral role in the delivery of healthcare. The importance is recognised of all stakeholders accessing good-quality information and reasoning, in order to clarify the argument for changing clinical practice. Such information must be credible and where possible evidence based to make the relative advantages clear. The impact that organisational culture has over successful integration can expedite or mitigate integration, so a culture of continuous improvement and stability of engaged stakeholders is vital. When stakeholders clearly understand the role that TECS can play in delivering care and acknowledge the need for continuous improvement in the way that care is delivered, they are energised and enabled to so that TECS integration is much more likely to happen.

References

1. Taylor K. *Connected Health: how digital technology is transforming health and social care.* London: Deloitte Centre for Health Solutions; 2015. Available at: www2.deloitte.com/content/dam/Deloitte/uk/Documents/life-sciences-health-care/deloitte-uk-connected-health-sm1.pdf

2. NHS England (NHSE). *NHS Five Year Forward View.* London: NHSE; 2014. Available at: www.england.nhs.uk/wp-content/uploads/2014/10/5yfv-web.pdf

3. Greenhalgh T, Robert G, Macfarlane F *et al.* Diffusion of innovations in service organisations: systematic review and recommendations. *Millbank Q.* 2004; **82**(4): 581–629.

4. The King's Fund. *Cultural Assessment Tool.* London: The King's Fund; n.d. Available at: www.kingsfund.org.uk/leadership/collective-leadership/how-we-can-work-you-develop-collective-leadership

5. NHSE. *Technology Enabled Care Services (TECS).* London: NHSE; 2015. Available at: www.england.nhs.uk/ourwork/qual-clin-lead/tecs/

6. Cruickshank J with Beer G, Winpenny E *et al. Healthcare Without Walls: a framework for delivering telehealth at scale.* London: 2020Health.org; 2010. Available at: www.2020health.org/dms/2020health/downloads/reports/2020telehealthLOW.pdf

7. Chambers R, O'Connell P, Chambers C. *Clinician's CPD Programme for Digital Healthcare.* Stoke-on-Trent: Digital Health Stoke-on-Trent; 2015. Available at: www.digitalhealthsot.nhs.uk/index.php/clinicians-learning-centre/cpd-programme

8. Szulanski G. *Sticky Knowledge: barriers to knowledge in the firm.* London: Sage; 2003.

9. Buchanan D, Fitzgerald L. The best practices puzzle: why are new methods contained and not spread? In: Buchanan D, Fitzgerald L, Ketley D, editors. *The Sustainability and Spread of Organizational Change: modernizing healthcare.* Oxford: Routledge; 2007. pp. 41–59.

10. Department of Health (DH). *Innovation Health and Wealth: accelerating adoption and diffusion in the NHS.* London: DH; 2011.

11. Department of Health (DH). *Whole System Demonstrator Programme.* London: DH; 2011. Available at: www.gov.uk/government/publications/whole-system-demonstrator-programme-headline-findings-december-2011

12. www.simple.uk.net

13. NHS England. *The* Forward View *into Action.* London: NHSE; 2014. Available at: www.england.nhs.uk/wp-content/uploads/2014/12/forward-view-plning.pdf

14. NHSE. *Strategic Planning Resources for Commissioners.* London: NHSE; 2015. Available at: www.england.nhs.uk/ourwork/qual-clin-lead/tecs/strategic-planning/

15. Gorst S, Armitage C, Coates L; University of Sheffield and Manchester. *Mainstreaming Assisted Living Technologies: patient acceptance.* Sheffield: University of Sheffield; n.d. Available at: http://malt.group.shef.ac.uk/patient-acceptance/patient-acceptance/

16. Mainstreaming Assisted Living Technologies (MALT). *Telehealth Acceptance Measure to Assess Patient Motivation in the use of Telehealth: V1.* Sheffield: Univeristy of Sheffield MALT; 2014. Available at: http://malt.group.shef.ac.uk/assets/files/MALT%20TAM%20Final.pdf

Chapter 14

Including technology in the delivery of person-centred, integrated care

Dr Ruth Chambers

Integrated working is central to all plans to transform health and social care services. All related strategies aim to deliver more efficient, enhanced quality and more patient-focused care. Such strategies will only succeed with collaborative working across sectors and care settings to deliver integrated services. So this needs a change of culture – not just structure and processes alone – to achieve the outcomes everyone wants. To help make that change of culture happen in your local health economy you need to:

- communicate plans to everyone involved in delivery and receipt of care – by every communication means you can think of, to every group of people affected, in a planning cycle where feedback influences ongoing service transformation
- relay the sense of purpose of the change in ways that match with workforce priorities
- take steady steps forward, with much consultation and increasing commitment, rather than leap too fast to goals that are regarded as irrelevant by most of the workforce who'll be delivering the changed services
- enable everyone to work together – during the service reconfiguration, by learning together, supporting new ways of teamworking etc.

What is person-centred care?

In essence person-centred care is simply:

- the right care for the person's (or carer's) needs and preferences, delivered with dignity, compassion, sensitivity and respect, at the right time and place, with due regard to the person's age and any cognitive impairment.

In addition, it is:

- holistic care that includes physical, mental, emotional, spiritual and social aspects and the person's own perspective and experiences – as appropriate
- shared care: informed, value based, preference sensitive, agreed between person (and carer or family if appropriate) and care professional
- safe: with informed decision making balancing potential benefits and risks where there are options for different routes and modes of delivery of care
- designed and evaluated with public, community and patient input and feedback
- proactive and inclusive of health promotion as well as primary, secondary and tertiary prevention
- integral to a quality improvement culture in health and social care.[1]

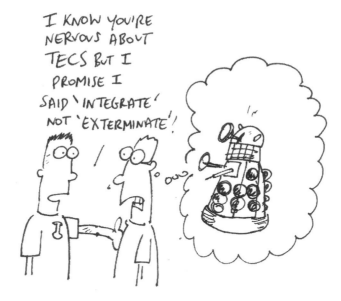

How can we make integrated care happen effectively with technology enabled care services (TECS)?

It is challenging for health and social care professionals working in different organisations and in a range of care settings to coordinate care management for a particular patient or service user that is underpinned by TECS. Who will pay for the technology equipment, who will set it up or maintain it, who will take responsibility if there is an abnormal reading or texted response – and when?

'Integrated care working' features in all health economies' strategies for provision of care, especially in relation to frail and complex patients who are the highest service users. It's one thing to adopt high-level strategies; it's another thing to make their implementation happen consistently well at the front line, valuing quality and safety of individual patients and service users.

'Integrated care' is defined or understood in different ways. It may be regarded as an intervention such as case management or care coordination. Or it may be viewed as a 'complex strategy to innovate and implement long-lasting change in the way services in the health and social care sectors are delivered'.[2] Principles for integrated care agreed on a national basis across health and social care[3,4] include:

- enable integrated care to develop quickly and at scale
- put patients and service users at the heart of care
- focus on patient or service user need
- timely and appropriate access to a network of services that aim to prevent ill health or offer alternatives to care
- common goals and governance systems
- delivery against national specified outcomes indicators.

There is much debate as to the evidence of benefits and cost-effectiveness of integrated care in general. But it is generally accepted that closer working between the NHS and social care which is designed to enhance productivity and deliver care in the right settings will help to address the substantive funding gap that the NHS faces in future with the increasing proportion of older, frail people in the populatiuon.[5-7] Effective integrated care will need to overcome the obstacles that inhibit care providers collaborating across organisational boundaries.[8,9]

Successful implementation of TECS will improve service quality or clinical outcomes, enhance patient experience and satisfaction, and reduce pressure on all health and social care services as patients or service users take more responsibility for their care or lifestyle habits in proactive ways. When such provision is designed to happen at all levels, that is, system level, organisational level, functional level, professional level, service level and personal level, then this creates and underpins integrated care.[6,10] Well coordinated care (e.g. post-discharge care) should significantly improve health and well-being outcomes.[6,11] Digital technology should give patients and clinicians a greater choice in respect of delivery of care, and adoption of self-care.[12]

Framework for extent and nature of integrated or person-centred care underpinning delivery of TECS by health and social care professionals in same or different settings[12]

Figure 14.1 captures the extent of responsibility for the digital interaction with patients or service users and their responsible one or more health and social care professionals working from different or the same settings in integrated ways.

1. **Shared real-time responsibility** by ≥2 clinicians or social workers, in different organisations or settings share same mode of technology for delivery of pre-agreed shared care plan of same patient or same condition at same treatment phase (named clinicians or social workers agree responsibility for specific points in patient pathway via care plan; organisations pre-agree the pathway and who pays for and supplies or monitors the technology).
2. **Shared sequential responsibility:** ≥2 clinicians or social workers, in different but interfacing organisations or settings; one **hands over** responsibility to the other for providing specific mode of digital delivery (same mode of technology or different) for continuing care of same patient or same condition via agreed care plan and pre-agreed shared clinical and social care protocols.
3. **Shared multidisciplinary protocol with one TECS operator:** ≥2 clinicians or social workers, of different disciplines, in same organisation or setting; sharing (delegated) responsibility for providing TECS directly (≥1 mode of technology) for continuing care of same patient or ≥1 conditions via agreed care plan and pre-agreed shared clinical or social care protocols.
4. **Self-contained delivery by individual professional:** TECS initiated and delivered by health or social care professional who updates other health or social care professionals or teams involved in the patient's care as appropriate (i.e. giving information rather than interactive decision making between professionals).
5. **Self-contained delivery by patient or service user:** TECS initiated and operated by person who updates their health or social care professionals or teams involved in their care (e.g. health app recording information relating to the person's health or lifestyle habits).

FIGURE 14.1 Framework for extent of responsibility for delivery of integrated or person-centred care via TECS by health and social care professionals[12]

Each level assumes that the patient or service user has given informed consent to participate; and that it may be one or more health conditions or one or more of a range of digital health modes of delivery provided or accessed.

EXAMPLE 14.1 Integrating care across the COPD patient pathway

A programme funded by West Midlands Academic Health Science Network (WMAHSN) is using Flo simple telehealth to underpin a model of integrated care. Five clinical commissioning groups (CCGs), an acute trust, a mental health trust, a community trust and community pharmacies all have licences to use Flo and have agreed in principle to deploy Flo across patient pathways. The integrated care services being developed, for example, include a patient with COPD being supported by a carer or social care via Flo and also by a GP practice or community team; but if their condition worsens and they need hospital admission, they can then be discharged early using the same Flo protocol as in the community or general practice, and return to their original accommodation where they are supported either by protocols aimed at the carer or the patient. The usual COPD protocol requires regular submission of sputum colour, temperature and breathing if appropriate, and oxygen saturation level measurements, plus a course of antibiotics and steroids to be available as rescue medication when necessary. The carer may help with this, or may need support for their own stress and anxiety, for which they can sign up for remote support via Flo. So the process of using Flo can involve social workers, nurses, GPs, hospital consultants, hospital and community pharmacists, as well as carers and patients.

Encouraging self-care[13]

Self-care is about people's attitudes and lifestyle, as well as what they can do to take care of themselves when they have a health problem. Supporting self-care is about increasing people's confidence and self-esteem, enabling them to take decisions about the sensible care of their health and avoiding triggering health problems. Although many people are already practising self-care to some extent, there is a great deal more that they can do.

The key is having health and social care professionals enthusiastically supporting self-care. All the team needs to be signed up to advocating self-care and finding ways for people with all kinds of health conditions to be able to self-care. This generates potential benefits in managing demands on health and social care services by patients and service users. So an integrated care approach encourages the effort to shift towards the self-care end of the continuum (*see* Figure 14.2).

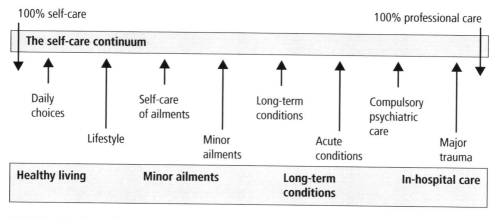

FIGURE 14.2 The self-care continuum

To promote effective self-care, commissioners and providers and frontline health and social care professionals must see and understand the patient or service user's perspective, learn to manage change and adopt the various self-care support described in Figure 14.3. To make self-care work both the public and professionals need knowledge and information (of facts and of where to find information), skills and motivation so that people are empowered to take a more active self-care role in maintaining or improving their health.

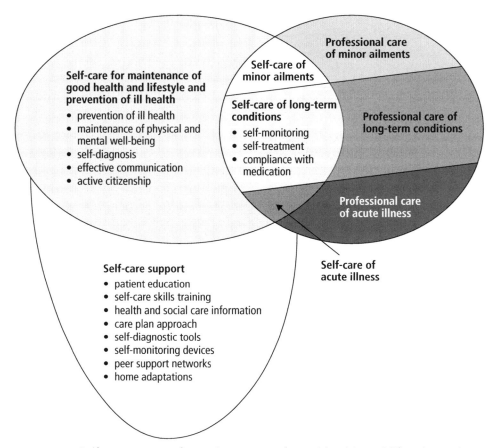

FIGURE 14.3 Self-care support for maintenance of good health and lifestyle, and prevention and care of ill health (courtesy: Ayesha Dost, Department of Health)[13]

TECS are a driver for self-care, and integrated working as a form of delivery of TECS features widely in the many chapters of this book, and neither can be considered in isolation.

EXAMPLE 14.2 Using TECS to create 'virtual wards'

The virtual wards trialled by Healthcare at Home of East Staffordshire have created the equivalent of 379 virtual beds. The wards are set up to allow multidisciplinary healthcare teams to monitor patients' bodily parameters relevant to their health conditions and state using a range of wireless vital signs monitors that connect with a tablet computer via Bluetooth. Sensors include blood pressure cuffs, blood glucose meters, pulse oximeters, heart rate monitors, and weight and body fat scales. The tablet then connects with a cloud computing system over the Internet so that the various readings of these vital signs can be triaged using predictive algorithms to detect any trends giving early indication of deterioration that can be actively managed to reduce likelihood of hospital (re)admission.

www.newscientist.com/living_health

FAQs

Q1 What is needed to make integrated health and social care really happen?

A. The elements that are vital for an integrated system of health and social services to succeed include quality measurement and data sharing tools to track outcomes and exchange information.[5] So then we might unlock such data, making them more easily available at the point of care and making them actionable. Then we can integrate care across a person's morbidities, providers and treatment plans.

Q2. Have TECS a role in enhancing patient safety in the delivery of integrated health and social care?

A. Very much so. TECS can support the evolution of a patient safety culture with more likely patient adherence to pre-agreed shared management plans, and better communication between clinicians and carers in different settings or between clinician and patient. Technology should be able to replace error-prone manual methods of delivery, which favour specific patients, with TECS that are automated and objective. If it was more obvious too where there was workforce capacity within the local health and social care system, patients could be directed that way more readily.

References

1. Chambers R, Hughes R, Parker C *et al*. *Our WMAHSN Manifesto for Person-Centred Care (PCC)*. Birmingham: West Midlands Academic Health Science Network; 2015. Available at: http://wmahsn.org/storage/resources/documents/WMAHSN_manifesto_for_Person_Centred_Care.pdf
2. Nolte E, Pitchforth E. *What is the Evidence on the Economic Impacts of Integrated Care?* Policy Summary 11. Copenhagen: World Health Organization Regional Office for Europe for the European Observatory on Health Systems and Policies; 2014. Available at: www.euro.who.int/__data/assets/pdf_file/0019/251434/What-is-the-evidence-on-the-economic-impacts-of-integrated-care.pdf
3. National Voices. *Principles for Integrated Care*. London: National Voices; 2014. Available at: www.nationalvoices.org.uk/
4. Age UK. *Agenda for Later Life: policy priorities for active ageing*. London: Age UK; 2012. Available at: www.ageuk.org.uk

5. McGinnis T, Crawford M, Somers S. *A State Policy Framework for Integrating Health and Social Services.* Commonwealth Fund Issue Brief pub. 1757. Vol. 14. New York, NY: The Commonwealth Fund; 2014. Available at: www.commonwealthfund.org

6. NHS Confederation and Local Government Association. *All Together Now: making integration happen.* London: NHS Confederation; 2014. Available at: www.nhsconfed.org

7. Monitor. *Closing the NHS Funding Gap: how to get better value health care for patients.* London: Monitor; 2013. Available at: www.gov.uk/government/uploads/system/uploads/attachment_data/file/284044/ClosingTheGap091013.pdf

8. Petch A. *Insights 24: delivering integrated care and support.* Glasgow: Institute for Research and Innovation in Social Services; 2014. Available at: www.iriss.org.uk

9. Graham C, Killpack C, Raleigh V *et al. Options Appraisal on the Measurement of People's Experiences of Integrated Care.* Oxford: Picker Institute Europe; 2013. Available at: www.pickereurope.org

10. Goodwin N, Dixon A, Anderson G *et al. Providing Integrated Care for Older People with Complex Needs: lessons from seven international case studies.* London: The King's Fund; 2014. Available at: www.kingsfund.org.uk

11. NHS England (NHSE). *Safe, Compassionate Care for Frail Older People using an Integrated Care Pathway: practical guidance for commissioners, providers and nursing, medical and allied health professional leaders.* South Horley: NHSE; 2014.

12. Chambers R *et al. Tackling Telehealth 2: how to develop integrated care through the implementation of TECS.* London: *Inside Commissioning*; 2015. Available at: www.digitalhealthsot.nhs.uk/index.php/clinicians-learning-centre/resources/documents/?task=document.viewdoc&id=37

13. Chambers R, Wakley G, Blenkinsopp A. *Supporting Self Care in Primary Care.* Abingdon: Radcliffe Publishing; 2006.

Part Three

Moving digital healthcare on

Chapter 15

Learning about technology enabled care services: so improving uptake

Dr Ruth Chambers

Learning about technology enabled care services (TECS) and being capable of deploying the various modes of delivery are not about education and training alone. They are about developing and utilising the skills, knowledge and abilities of all the staff in your organisation or team to ensure optimum, safe usage. You'll need to ensure that services continue to meet the needs of patients, new service developments and policy changes. Your organisational or team learning should be a process of continual improvement and innovation – an ongoing cycle of action and reflection followed by revision of your approach.

Sorry, but learning how to use technology is not an option

Most organisations or teams have their share of reluctant learners. These will include very experienced staff members with long service records, people who are considering retirement or those who are not ambitious and are satisfied with their current role or level of responsibility. The challenge is to engage these individuals, as their contribution in the team or to delivery is important to the overall effectiveness and productivity of your service and pathways. So these reluctant learners need to accept that learning about types of digital delivery and upskilling them to select and action TECS are inherent to their continuing role and not an optional extra.

Learning styles

Everyone has their preferred learning styles. Anyone introducing a change such as new ways of delivering care via TECS needs to vary their styles and offer a range of modes of training, so that it meets every learner's needs and there is something of interest for everyone.

Honey and Mumford described four learning styles, as follows.[1,2]

Activists: like to be fully involved in new experiences, are open-minded, will try anything once, thrive on the challenge of new experiences but soon get bored and want to go on to the next challenge. Activists learn best through new experiences, short activities and situations where they can be centre stage (chairing meetings, leading discussions), and when allowed to generate new ideas, and have a go at new things or brainstorm ideas.

Reflectors: like to stand back, think about things thoroughly and collect a lot of information before coming to a conclusion. They are cautious, take a back seat in meetings and discussions, adopt a low profile and appear tolerant and unruffled. Reflectors learn best from situations where they are allowed to watch and think about activities before taking action. They carry out research first of all, review evidence, have produced carefully constructed reports and can reach decisions in their own time.

Theorists: like to adapt and integrate observations into logical maps and models, using step-by-step processes. They tend to be perfectionists, and are detached, analytical and objective. They reject anything that is subjective, flippant and lateral thinking in nature. Theorists learn best from activities where there are plans, maps and models to describe what is going on. They prefer to take time to explore the methodology and work with structured situations with a clear purpose, when they are offered complex situations to understand and are intellectually stretched.

Pragmatists: like to try out ideas, theories and techniques to see if they work in practice. They will act quickly and confidently in relation to ideas that attract them and are impatient when others are ruminating and participating in endless discussions. They like solving problems and making practical decisions, responding to problems as a challenge. Pragmatists learn best when there is an obvious link between the subject and their roles. They enjoy trying out techniques with coaching and feedback, practical issues, real problems to solve and when they are given the immediate chance to implement what they have learnt.

EXERCISE 15.1

Once you're more aware of the learning style that matches your approach, make your learning plan for TECS and discuss with your mentor or line manager or local TECS lead, and find ways to take that forward, such as online, shadowing a TECS expert, trying a TECS pathway out for yourself etc.

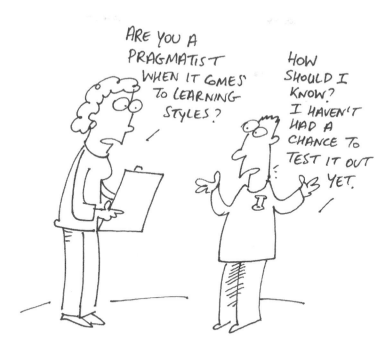

Partnership learning that is cross-boundary (e.g. acute and primary care settings), and cross-cultural between partner organisations (e.g. voluntary sector and NHS) will help to drive the implementation of TECS on a wide scale. In complex environments where professions, organisations and even public, voluntary and private sector organisations work together, the obvious thing is also to learn together about TECS and the provision of person-centred care.

Learning in partnership with other organisations may require a different mindset, being willing to share organisational information (e.g. using the NHS number to identify individual patients), developing trust-based relationships and sharing costs and risks. So this will require the NHS and other organisations to work together in non-traditional ways. Everyone should know what the purpose of their organisation is in relation to their shared vision with other organisations or teams with whom they integrate care, and deliver TECS at all levels in the organisation. Individual members of staff will need a clear sense of direction to ensure that they all work towards common goals and understand what is expected from them as individuals and their team. The organisation will need a matrix of leaders with responsibility for developing vision, strategic planning, organisational performance, redesign and extension of services, service quality and workforce development – for synchronised delivery of TECS to work effectively. There should be opportunities for two-way communication. Communication between management and staff should not be a token gesture but should have real value; individual members of staff need to have ownership over the way in which they work and learn too.

Being more effective at work with TECS

Motivated and skilled staff should be able to use TECS effectively to:

1. manage an ever increasing workload – by better deployment of staff skills to deliver care remotely
2. reduce vacancies and staff turnover – by boosting job satisfaction
3. develop special interests – that lead to more patients or service users being treated at home or with shared care between clinicians and carers in different settings
4. create shorter patient waiting times – with more efficient use of staff skills
5. achieve more personalised person-centred care
6. establish a more flexible and responsive workforce – staff who are more adaptable in response to patient demand (e.g. initiating remote care by Skype)
7. provide more proactive care and prompt response to problems as they happen (e.g. with telehealth)
8. set up shared learning across and between organisations; between different staff groups and disciplines (e.g. with a closed Facebook group)
9. improve communication between professionals in different teams; and clinicians with patients or service users (e.g. by multidisciplinary team meetings via encrypted video links).

Getting clinicians or social workers using TECS

It shouldn't be a big leap for professionals who use digital modes in their personal lives (mobile phone apps or Skype) to also use digital delivery in the care that they provide.

So if you're a team leader or champion of TECS, relay the following headlines to your peers or other staff.

- Consider using a digital mode of delivery as routine when reviewing someone's need for care or care plan – mainstreaming digital delivery of care. Include questions about a patient's or service user's technical capability or ownership of technology in an assessment of a person's care needs:
  —Do you use the Internet?
  —Do you have a mobile phone? What type?
  —Do you want follow-on care by digital delivery?
- Push education: make people (clinicians or patient) aware of what's available or how to do it (easily).
- Cite good and memorable case studies: set up a library so that whoever is the 'audience' can relate to others' experiences.
- Encourage new models of assessment, with the same care planning template in different health and social care settings.
- Give good examples of successful use of TECS for patients or service users

– qualitative reports might include how TECS improved their personal or working lives; reassurance that came from text reminders to reinforce care plans or interventions.

- Describe good examples of successful use of TECS by health and social care professionals – qualitative reports describing increased productivity as patients managed by telehealth liberate more time for people who need face-to-face consultations; or quantitative evaluation showing NHS cost savings from avoided healthcare usage.
- Combat prejudice – about innovation etc.
- Promote easy to use protocols – seen as accredited, safe, promoting consistent quality, so these can just be adopted (or adapted by health or social care professionals for their setting or individual receiver).
- Emphasise that they should take on TECS gradually and learn to use different modes of delivery of care in comfortable ways with support from others familiar with that TECS.
- Anticipate obstacles and ways to overcome challenges – with case studies.
- Discuss automation versus interactivity – getting the balance right (for user); and fit for purpose.
- Aid professionals to use TECS to look after themselves – or help carers to do that; maybe an accredited health app might help them to combat migraines or back pain.
- Use 'league tables' so that areas or teams sited where there is a void of digital care usage are 'shamed' by the high user areas.

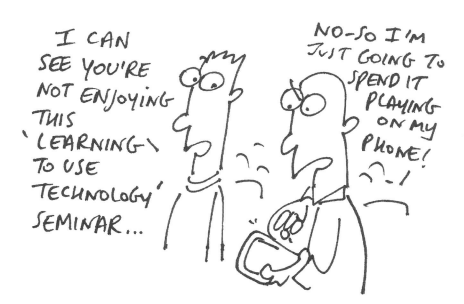

- Push the message – real empowerment of patients means trusting them, sharing meaningful information with them, expecting patients to undertake agreed interventions.
- Use the right content in any protocol that defines the use of TECS; ensure the tone of the messages is right, personalise to the user (if easy to do).

Showcasing evidence

You'll learn a lot about TECS if you try out a type of technology in your everyday work, and collect evidence about the application – what happens, how patients or service users benefit, what the consequence costs are, how much smoother (or otherwise) your delivery of care is and how everyone involved rates the service you provide. So:

- carry out the pilot – evaluate it in a way that you can generalise to other patients or service users, or other team members
- illustrate cost savings (e.g. time spent with patient or service user as proxy measure of cost) to colour future business plans so you can ensure that plans for a wider rollout are pitched right
- network with other organisations or networks using TECS successfully or innovatively – such as Academic Health Science Networks; share good practice and lessons learned
- gather all perspectives – user, health or social professionals, managers (quality, access, usefulness, efficiency and productivity)
- note any reductions in travel time – greener delivery of care as well as your liberation from unnecessary home visits
- select an app approved for use in health and social care (if that is the type of technology you're piloting) from the NHS library apps database so that it is regarded as 'safe'
- consider setting up a Facebook group (for patients/service users or clinicians) – so you can share stories about the use of TECS.

Join in a more substantive evaluation locally to compare costs and effort between usual ways of delivery of care versus more productive ways via digital delivery; target high cost areas of care such as people with severe COPD where there is good evidence for the benefits of digital care.[3–6]

Being flexible

You'll need to work with individual patients or service users to find a method (or two!) of digital delivery that suits their needs and preferences as well as going with what is available or affordable. You might make an intelligent decision for automated messaging or interaction that is focused on the purpose, and triggers the patient or service user to take action.

What to try

Maybe try:

- two different types of TECS, such as two of telehealth, Skype, app (that allows free dispatch of photos etc.)
- stepping up and down the level of clinical management for an individual patient with more or less intense delivery of digital care and associated treatment
- including family members in making the regular interaction with digital mode of delivery happen; they might be able to interact (e.g. respond regularly on behalf of person with dementia; lend their relative their smartphone)
- integrating delivery of care between two or more settings (e.g. health and social care; clinician and patient)
- using a landline connection rather than a mobile phone – if that suits the user
- advising the service user what can be bought or used by an individual from bargain retail stores to help keep them safe
- setting up TECS so that specific individual staff members in a team or those providing integrated care can access the TECS records of an individual (by the individual's signed consent)
- giving a demonstration of your use of TECS to teams of professionals elsewhere; this will help to build your confidence and know-how.

Wide-ranging local learning programme requirements

Any wide-ranging local learning programme for TECS should have:

1. *Transparency* – who can undertake the learning opportunities (e.g. staff at all levels and with a range of roles).
2. *Equity* – aiming to deliver digital care to a wide range of patients or service users rather than focus on particular types of professionals.
3. *Comprehensiveness* – support for all health and social care staff, with or without existing professional qualifications.
4. *Responsiveness* – adapt the learning programme to support development of new skills as requirements and availability of TECS change and the workforce develops.
5. *Integration* – care staff of different disciplines should learn together in collaborative ways; with new models of delivery of care as work-based teams.
6. *Partnership* – health, social care, private and voluntary sectors should work together to deliver TECS, so ways and scope of learning should match this.
7. *Flexibility* –
   - people should be able to step on and off learning, accumulating credits

if that's appropriate; to make intermittent upskilling more viable to develop their career potential throughout their working lives
- bring education to the teams where they work.
8. *Viability* – encourage real learning based on clinical and social care practice, not theory
9. *An outcomes focus* – delivering tangible outcomes; thinking and planning in terms of health gains (from commissioners', managers', clinicians' and patients' perspectives) rather than improvements in structures and systems.

EXAMPLE 15.1 Frailty toolkit training

Digital technology can be used to enhance health and social care professionals' learning by bringing professionals together from different settings to learn together and experience a virtual reality simulation exercise, for delegates to appreciate what everyday life is like if you are yourself frail. Take a look at the participants' experiences of using the app on: www.pcdc.org.uk/admin/resources/november-2015-frailty-toolkit-newsletter.pdf

---

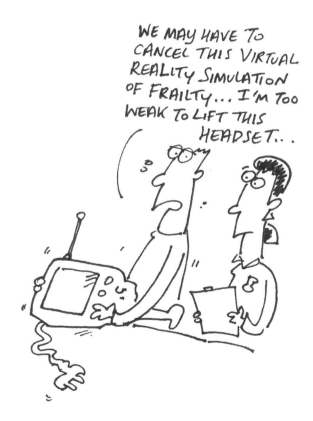

Leading service redesign – maybe by positive dissonance

Whatever role you have in the NHS or social care, you can contribute to a service development or redesign that includes TECS. If you are a team leader, or clinician, social worker or manager you can make a difference. Find out how you can develop a successful business case (*see* Chapter 11) or engage with others who have influence or authority. Learn from Example 15.2 how you might achieve change. Positive dissonance is a useful personality trait or behaviour – that you can learn to adopt or adapt so that you facilitate or lead changes that will have a real impact on improving the quality and effectiveness of care delivered. If you're an achiever you have a moral responsibility to use your talents and skills to generate improvements in health and social care for the population, don't you?

EXAMPLE 15.2   A real achiever: his tips on what builds credibility and success

Neil Smith shared his insights into how to be a top achiever when he received his honorary doctorate from Keele University, which was awarded in recognition of his global achievements. He urged driven individuals (like himself) who are intending to make positive change happen to do the following.

1. Maintain your integrity and credibility – and others will trust you to lead the way or provide them with solutions to their problems.
2. Keep your promises and commitments (or, if impossible, agree new outcomes and provide more value).
3. Stand up for what's right. Don't be too timid to speak out even if you're a junior member of the team. Your persona is about who you are and what you stand for.
4. Try your hardest to complete your work plan – stick at it if it is worth doing.
5. Don't be timid about asking for what you want to improve your delivery of work tasks or change; you won't get that extra help otherwise, and others can't read your mind!
6. Offer doable solutions rather than complaining about problem issues; don't take 'no' for the final answer.
7. Be two or three (or four or five!) steps ahead of others. Anticipate the various activities you need to complete proactively so that you've got the necessary elements in place to achieve goals when others start planning the outcomes they want – or announce grants or other funds you can bid for.
8. Build your networks and relationships with others – you never know who's going to be 'useful' to you in future (or you 'useful' to them) even when you have a different role or work base. Maintain a reasonable level of communication and contact.
9. Enjoy your interactions with others. Even if you're not a super-sociable person,

you can exploit your personality traits to communicate and engage in ways that suit you.

10. Think widely – and out of the box; use creative (but realistic) thinking.
11. Learn to listen to others; a critical friend can really improve your strategy, plan, report or options appraisal – inputting their expertise and ideas (which you might accept depending on the constraints and opportunities that you're aware of).
12. Market yourself and your skills and experience – don't be shy; use Twitter, websites and online platforms to highlight your achievements and what you can offer.
13. Balance your work and family life, making time for friends and hobbies – oh, and a healthy lifestyle.
14. Be happy – so you work productively and effectively over time.

EXERCISE 15.2   Learning to plan for the future delivery of TECS in your organisation or team

Plan how you will get your envisaged TECS pathway set up. First complete Table 15.1 (Exercise 15.2a) to draft the plan from which you will draw the strategy and implementation plan that you will continue to evolve to take to your board or manager to endorse. Then alongside that programme plan complete Exercise 15.2b as to how you will find the resources and create the infrastructure for dependable delivery, and Exercise 15.2c to plan the training and upskilling needed. You should now be ready to complete the business plan template of your organisation as Exercise 15.2d.

Exercise 15.2a: Complete Table 15.1

TABLE 15.1 Programme plan: activities and tasks of your intended programme to introduce TECS in delivery of care in your workplace

	Timescale (days, weeks or months)									
Activities and tasks										
Develop justification and vision for TECS applications										
Search for any similar use of TECS in same or different setting, and type of users; gain evidence of benefits from others' applications										
Identify key stakeholders and engage them as allies with shared purpose, priorities and foci for TECS										
Create strategy or business plan; share drafts and revise including others' views, building allies										

	Timescale (days, weeks or months)									
Submit strategy to board (other) for agreement; modify with its critique or resubmit – as appropriate										
Implement a communication plan for staff involvement, team briefing etc.										
Develop relevant policies, protocols, clinical governance or information governance etc. and attach when approved										
Integration of planning and learning										
Corporate planning cycle begins: establish organisational goals and priorities (e.g. *see* SWOT exercise in Chapter 9)										
Implementation plan: infrastructure and resource matrix										
Develop learning and training plan: skills escalator, core programmes, shared programme etc.										
Integration of learning and key functions: clinical governance, risk management, complaints, public and patient involvement										
Develop and action evaluation process – capturing variety perspectives (outcome data, people's experiences and views)										
Regular review process to check progress and capture learning, gaps etc.										
Publish report for sponsor or general public (as appropriate)										

Exercise 15.2b

Plan how you will create your infrastructure for a TECS pathway and find the resources needed – check that all elements of Table 15.2 are in your proposed business case and delivery plan.

This exercise will help you to assess the readiness of your organisation's or team's infrastructure in the development of a wide-scale learning programme for all staff members.

TABLE 15.2 Learning to plan proactively for sufficient resources to complete the implementation of the digital mode of delivery of care

Infrastructure or resources	Elements
Documentation	Policy, protocols, standards, operating procedures, privacy impact assessment, information governance etc.
Location	Physical location, available space, training facilities etc.
Money	Protected or identified funding, budgets, bids, grants etc.
Expertise	Skills, knowledge, capability, competence within or without the organisation or team, training and education provision

Infrastructure or resources	Elements
People	Appropriately trained and available staff, staff hours, coverage for training etc.
Materials	Equipment, technology equipment, TECS protocols, training resources, supplies, provisions etc.
Information technology (IT)	Hardware, software, networks, Internet capability, library facilities, knowledge management systems
Communication	Communication flows, mechanisms, e.g. newsletter, team briefing, user involvement, community, media and press
Planning	Planning groups, project management capability and strategic planning meetings, links to managers and frontline staff

Exercise 15.2c

Plot your organisation's or team's resources by ticking where there are identified resources available or inserting a cross where there are none in Table 15.3. By identifying these gaps you can begin to build an action plan of the next steps to ensure that there are easily available learning and upskilling opportunities for all, in your development of delivery of TECS.

TABLE 15.3 Proactive learning plan for sufficient resources to complete the training needed to underpin the implementation of digital modes of delivery of care

Study leave or protected learning time initiatives and incentives	
Policy for clinical supervision	
Quality assurance for providers	
Systematic evaluation	
Clinical governance or information governance monitoring	
Risk management processes	
Partnership learning with other organisations	
Curriculum development with universities, colleges or online providers	

Exercise 15.2d: Complete the business plan

You or a team member will need to complete the business plan. Look at Chapter 11 for the worked example – but better still find out what template your organisation uses so that you are completing all the sections that will be necessary for your organisation to support your delivery plan.

Push for a continuous improvement culture

Everyone has their part to play in continuing quality improvement in their work setting – whether they are a care professional, manager, administrator or leader.

So you need a focused mindset for continuing improvement as well as an organisational culture. Key elements will be:

- preserving safety and effectiveness of care provided
- problem solving – on an individual patient or service user basis or for a recurring organisational issue; getting to the root of a problem and redressing it satisfactorily
- data analyses – interpreting how well the care provided matches the specification or standards pre-set, how well outcomes of delivery of care benchmark against other providers of similar care; with an associated action plan to address gaps in quality
- review of all key stages in delivery of a care pathway – what, how, where and when care is needed and by whom, synchronised across health and social care settings
- lean thinking – focusing on the quality of delivery required for individuals, minimising waste and unwarranted clinical or other variation.

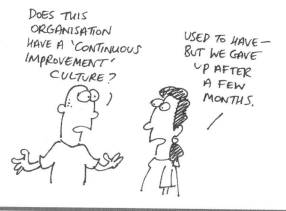

EXERCISE 15.3

Take a look at *The NHS Change Model*[1] which should give you more insights into how to lead sustainable change and service transformation, with there being an agreed shared purpose across health and care. You will then develop your approach in relation to the eight components of this model: shared purpose, leadership for change, spread of innovation, improvement methodology, rigorous delivery, transparent measurement, system drivers and engagement to mobilise.

Or you might adopt the *plan, do, study, act* (PDSA) cycle as your preferred improvement tool to make your envisaged change happen. Plan explicitly your (small) change; do what you have planned to do; study the expected outcomes and any that you did not expect; act on the results to modify and improve your service. If you start small, you've more chance of achieving what your vision set out, then building momentum as others can see the evidence of your improvement.

Significant event audit or analysis

Unless you're very lucky, something is likely to go wrong as you progress your strategy, implementation plan or delivery programme, even with great planning. You need to spot a significant event early, and analyse what's happened to learn from it, change the system or elements of the programme and get things back on track. A significant event might encompass any aspect of service delivery – operational, managerial and clinical – and the audit should be viewed as a constructive process that offers significant learning for a pan-organisational application of delivery of TECS. The process covers four basic stages:

1. Select the event you want to analyse in relation to digital delivery – maybe a service gap in overseeing technology-relayed responses from patients?
2. Gather the data needed; this might relate to clinical outcomes, or TECS usage, and will probably include patient or service user perspectives too.
3. Hold a meeting with everyone involved (e.g. health and social care professionals, managers) to analyse the significant event and agree on actions to minimise likelihood of recurrence.
4. Implement action and review the effects.

EXERCISE 15.4

Try completing a significant event audit or analysis using the template in Table 15.4. Discuss it with colleagues or your manager and take action as suggested in the section after this exercise.

TABLE 15.4 Checklist for significant event audit or analysis focused on particular delivery episode of digital care

Issues	Action	Results
How was the event managed initially?		
Who was involved?		
What were the positive things that occurred?		
Could anyone else have contributed to the event?		
How could they have contributed?		
What were the key factors that determined the outcome?		

Issues	Action	Results
Were there any interface issues?		
Were there any team issues?		
Follow-up arrangements		

Then draft and finalise your subsequent action plan.

- How and when will change be implemented?
- What action or policy decision will you take as a result of this audit or analysis?
- Who will be responsible for ensuring that this is done?
- When will the tasks be completed?
- When will you re-audit the relevant elements of the delivery of digital care?

Gauge the driving and restraining factors that will influence whether your digital delivery plan is likely to happen and be embedded in local services

You could try drawing up a force-field analysis of positive drivers and negative influences in the implementation or expansion of digital delivery of care by your organisation or team. Do it with all others involved in the planning or envisaged delivery.

Why you should use this approach: In order to help people to identify and focus on the positive and negative forces in their application of TECS and to gain an overview of the weighting of these factors.

EXERCISE 15.5

Draw up a force-field analysis which is laid out in a similar way to Table 15.5.

What to do: draw a horizontal or vertical line in the middle of a sheet of paper. Label one side 'positive' and the other side 'negative'. Draw arrows to represent individual positive drivers that motivate you or your team to use TECS or apply a particular type of digital delivery of care on one side of the line, and negative factors that demotivate you on the negative side of the line. The chunkiness and length of the arrows should represent the extent of the influence; that is, a short, narrow arrow will indicate that the positive or negative factor has a minor influence and a long, wide arrow a major effect.

How much time you should allow: up to an hour with ensuing discussion if you're doing this as a small group or team; longer to allow for subsequent action planning.

TABLE 15.5 Example of force-field analysis diagram: planning for digital delivery of care

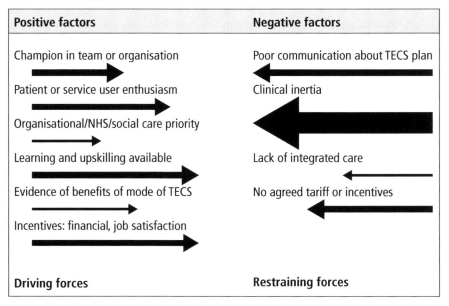

Positive factors	Negative factors
Champion in team or organisation	Poor communication about TECS plan
Patient or service user enthusiasm	Clinical inertia
Organisational/NHS/social care priority	
Learning and upskilling available	Lack of integrated care
Evidence of benefits of mode of TECS	No agreed tariff or incentives
Incentives: financial, job satisfaction	
Driving forces	**Restraining forces**

Then take an overview of the force field (if doing this on your own or as team group discussion) and consider if you are content with things as they are, or can think of ways to boost the positive side and minimise the negative factors.

Doing Exercise 15.5 should help you to realise whether a particular element is a positive or negative factor. For instance, you may realise upon reflection that time invested in setting up TECS is more than compensated for by time saved.

What to do next: make a personal or organisational action plan to create the situations and opportunities to boost the positive factors and minimise arrows on the negative side. Get someone else who knows your situation to review the force-field analysis you've drawn and spot any blind spots and if the positive and negative influences are in proportion.

Understanding key barriers to adoption of TECS

Evaluation of the use of TECS[8] has shown that, overall, satisfaction appeared optimal when patients were carefully selected for a particular protocol, when professional users were familiar with the system and the TECS programme addressed a problem or gap in previous methods of service delivery that had been identified by the clinicians using it. Some of the problems that professionals have are insufficient training or lack of knowledge about how to use the system and any problems with the local IT service. Such problems may reduce over time once routines and uses of the system become ingrained in everyday practice. Concern among professionals about patients' ability to use the technology may be unfounded; even those patients with little confidence in their ability to undertake the required activities actually can manage the technology in the end.[9]

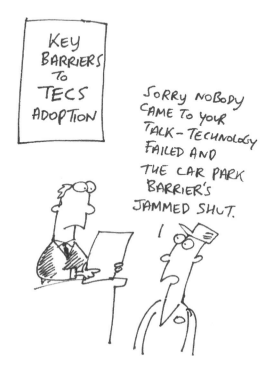

Professional users need to take a longer term view in investing time initially to become familiar with any new TECS system in order to provide a slicker, more accessible service in the future.

A systematic review of the literature[10] relating to frontline nursing staff's adoption of telehealth found that there is:

- ongoing difficulties in demonstrating evidence of benefit from telehealth and a lack of consistent and robust evaluation data
- confusion over who leads on telehealth implementation and how benefits can be realised over time
- staff uncertainty about telehealth limits adoption and acceptance, making it less likely that members offer telehealth to patients
- uncertainty too among potential patient users and their carers about the availability and value of telehealth
- no one business model that is appropriate for all service adoption and provision

- complexity in the implementation of telehealth in respect of commissioning, delivery, management and interconnectivity.

The reviewers recommended:

- improved and consistent evaluation when TECS are deployed, matched to the aims and needs of all involved
- enhanced understanding of the complexity and diversity of all stakeholders involved
- a greater recognition of the benefits of TECS in clinical practice
- TECS implementation is set up so that adoption is well supported in clinical practice
- greater recognition of the benefits of TECS by patients and service users which should then stimulate demand by the general public to try it
- business modelling to take into account the issues and challenges relating to TECS that need to be overcome to ensure sustainability of the model
- incorporating activities to mitigate against the complexity and challenges from operational, organisational and financial barriers in any TECS implementation plan.

EXERCISE 15.6

The reviewers have produced a freely available toolkit of resources for others to learn from their experience and knowledge.[10] Take a look at it and see if you can overcome any of the barriers that are obstructing the adoption or dissemination of TECS by your team, patient or service user groups or organisation.

Building your team

First: how motivated are they?

The best way to discover what motivates people is to ask them what they want or need in order to do a better job. Some will want more money, others more time, some more flexibility in their work schedule, others to take on new and more challenging roles.

Human nature makes people respond better to praise than punishment, so celebrate people's achievements. As for any kind of feedback, start with the positive and with the small things. The praise should come:

- immediately after the successful completion of part or all of a particular task
- from someone who knows what the task involved (not a remote committee)
- from an understanding of what the task involved.

EXERCISE 15.7

People are motivated by different things. Pick out some of the best motivators for fulfilling health or social care professionals' needs as listed below:

- interesting or useful work
- a sense of achievement
- responsibility
- opportunities for career progression or professional development
- gaining new skills or competences
- a sense of belonging to a healthcare organisation or practice team
- personal or written congratulations from a respected colleague or immediate superior
- public recognition
- announcement of success at team meetings
- recognising that the last job was well done and asking for an opinion of the next one
- providing specific and frequent feedback (positive first)
- providing information on how the task has affected the performance of the organisation or management of a patient
- encouragement to increase their knowledge and skills to do even better
- making time to listen to ideas, complaints or difficulties
- learning from mistakes and making visible changes.

Try to introduce these into your programme plan or to encourage colleagues' or team members' professional development.

Next strengthen your teamworking

EXERCISE 15.8

Good teamwork does not just happen. Take time out as a team away from the work-place to review how you are working together.

During a team away half-day when the team is reviewing progress or preparing to promote a new initiative, ask everyone in the team to complete the quiz below and rate their take on things:

There is good communication between colleagues at work	*usually / seldom / not at all*
There is good communication between managers and staff	*usually / seldom / not at all*
Team members' functions are clear	*usually / seldom / not at all*

Staff are proud to be working in your practice/unit	*usually / seldom / not at all*
Doctors/managers resolve staff problems	*usually / seldom / not at all*
Staff are treated with respect by clinicians and managers	*usually / seldom / not at all*
There is a person-friendly culture at work	*usually / seldom / not at all*
There are opportunities for staff for self-improvement	*usually / seldom / not at all*
Positive feedback about performance is the norm at work	*usually / seldom / not at all*
Staff are well trained for the tasks they are asked to do	*usually / seldom / not at all*
Team members' responsibilities are clear	*usually / seldom / not at all*
There is good leadership of the team	*usually / seldom / not at all*

Score: usually = 3, seldom = 1, not at all = 0.

Scores between 27 and 36: you have a well-functioning team

Scores between 24 and 15: look at your weak areas and make plans for improvements

Scores of 15 and below: as you have a long way to go, it may be best for you to consider using an external consultant to help facilitate team development

How it works (insight): everyone should have an equal chance of giving their perspective as to how the team is functioning. Completing the quiz independently allows everyone to be honest.

FAQs

Q1. So how do I learn about TECS and then get to set it up in my workplace?

A. Creating a TECS infrastructure at your workplace will need a change of culture and expectations of patients or service users and managers or professionals. Find other TECS enthusiasts and examples of where TECS works elsewhere and show that it is for everyday use by everyone working in health and social care; not just innovators using digital care. Get buy-in from everyone: operational managers and frontline staff as well as patients or service users.

Q2. How do I make this learning fit what's required for my professional continuing professional development (CPD)?

A. Look for ideas at www.networks.nhs.uk/nhs-networks/simple-telehealth/cpd-programme for the approach developed for Flo simple telehealth when it was initially rolled out across the UK. Try undertaking the CPD outline programme with any kind of digital mode of delivery of care.

Q3. What improves the chances of a successful project happening?

A. You need to get the right people involved from the start of the project – in thinking it through; then later doing it. You need clear aims that capture the initial situation and issues that are achievable with links to other stakeholders' priorities and strategies. You need to measure achievements and not just activities or processes. You should involve patients or service users from the beginning in designing the project, changing the service and defining success criteria and expected outcomes. And you should communicate all these elements well to everyone involved on a regular basis.

References

1. Garcarz W, Chambers R, Ellis S. *Make your Healthcare Organisation a Learning Organisation.* Abingdon: Radcliffe Medical Press; 2003.
2. Honey P, Mumford A. *Using your Learning Styles.* Maidenhead: Peter Honey Publications; 1986.
3. Udsen FW, Hejlesen O, Ehlers LH. A systematic review of the cost and cost-effectiveness of telehealth for patients suffering from chronic obstructive pulmonary disease. *J Telemed Telecare.* 2014; **20**(4): 212–20. Available at: www.ncbi.nlm.nih.gov/pubmed/24803277
4. Cruz J, Brooks D, Marques A. Home telemonitoring in COPD: a systematic review of methodologies and patients' adherence. *Int J Med Inform.* 2014; **83**(4): 249–63. Available at: www.ncbi.nlm.nih.gov/pubmed/24529402
5. Farmer A, Toms C, Hardinge M *et al.* Self-management support using an Internet-linked tablet computer (the EDGE platform)-based intervention in chronic obstructive pulmonary disease: protocol for the EDGE-COPD randomised controlled trial. *BMJ Open.* 2014; **4**(1): e004437. Available at: www.ncbi.nlm.nih.gov/pubmed/24401729
6. Voncken-Brewster V, Tange H, Moser A *et al.* Integrating a tailored e-health self-management application for chronic obstructive pulmonary disease patients into primary care: a pilot study. *BMC Fam Pract.* 2014; **15**: 4. Available at: www.ncbi.nlm.nih.gov/pubmed/24400676
7. NHS Sustainable Improvement Team. *Change Model.* Leeds: NHS Sustainable Improvement Team; 2013. Available at: www.nhsiq.nhs.uk/capacity-capability.aspx
8. Cottrell E, Cox T, Chambers R *et al.* Patient and professional user experiences of simple telehealth for hypertension, medication reminders and smoking cessation: a service evaluation. *BMJ Open.* 2015; **5**(3) e007270. Available at: http://bmjopen.bmj.com/content/5/3/e007270.full?keytype=ref&ijkey=iSJSZ2lP6qlocrO
9. Williams V, Price J, Hardinge M *et al.* Using a mobile health application to support self-management in COPD: a qualitative study. *Br J Gen Pract.* 2014; **64**(624): e392–400.
10. The MALT Study Consortium. *Overcoming the Barriers to Mainstreaming Assisted Living Technologies: summary research report.* Sheffield: University of Sheffield Mainstreaming Assisted Living Technologies (MALT); 2014. Available at: http://malt.group.shef.ac.uk/assets/files/MALT%20Final%20Summary%20Report%20Nov%202014.pdf

Chapter 16

Evaluation of technology enabled care services

Dr Lizzie Cottrell, Dr Ruth Chambers

Use of technology enabled care services (TECS) is well justified and appropriate if the benefits outweigh the costs (including time, financial and burden) to patients, professionals or services. Depending upon the aim of the TECS the benefits may not be explicit, although some of the costs may be. Evaluation is a tool that can be used to demonstrate the benefits, costs and value of the service from the perspectives of patients or service users, care professionals and managers. Unfortunately, many modes of technology have not been evaluated when

---

EXAMPLE 16.1 What is sleep-E-head?

The hypothetical service, sleep-E-head, was designed to improve sleep through mobile phone-based educational messages, an individualised treatment plan with goals set by the patient with support of a practice nurse and the use of a mobile phone application to monitor the quantity and quality of sleep and transmit this to a central server when a sensor is placed on the patient's head. It was introduced by a clinical commissioning group (CCG) after its prescribing lead noted a recent steady increase in the prescribing of hypnotic medications.

The aims of sleep-E-head were to:

1. increase patients' quality of sleep
2. increase patients' quantity of sleep
3. reduce hypnotic drug prescriptions across the CCG.

---

they have been produced or adopted in service provision, even though the providers may have collected some outcome data through tracking and self-reporting.

This chapter will describe what types of evaluation and audit there are, add a little more about why evaluation is important, and how you can get started in evaluating a TECS service. To contextualise the information contained within the chapter, an approach to a hypothetical technology enabled care service, sleep-E-head, is described throughout the chapter (*see* Example 16.1).

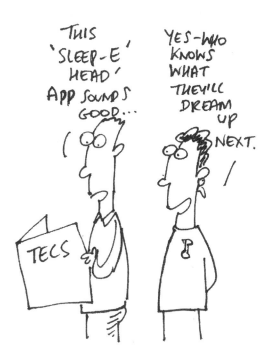

What is evaluation?

Evaluation may refer to service evaluation, the process of determining the standard to which your service is reaching.[1] Included patients are involved in your evaluation of the service because they and their responsible care professional agreed that this would be the service that best meets their needs; that is, they would have been involved in using the service whether you chose to evaluate it or not.

What is clinical audit?

Clinical audit compares the delivery of services against predetermined standards as a quality improvement process. Aspects of the structure, processes and outcomes of healthcare are selected and systematically evaluated against explicit criteria. Change in service provision should underpin the clinical audit process where gaps in care delivery are found at individual professional, team or service level. Then further monitoring or a repeated clinical audit cycle is used to confirm improvement in healthcare delivery.[2]

The steps of the audit cycle are:

* prioritise and select the topic of the audit
* set objectives: relating to the reasons why the audit is being carried out
* review the literature and agree the criteria and standards for that topic that you think are reasonable
* design the way in which you will do the audit
* collect the data and look at them
* feedback the findings; meet with colleagues or your team to discuss the findings and determine the reasons for the results
* make a timetabled action plan to implement any changes that are needed
* review your standards – should you keep the standards you previously set or are they unrealistic or not challenging enough?
* re-audit – creating successive audit cycles.

Why evaluate?

The benefits of evaluating services to determine performance have been underlined by key healthcare bodies such as Health Education England[3] and The King's Fund.[4] Proving the worth of services is important to demonstrate good use of (public) money and also to contribute to the evidence base, so that others can learn from your experiences, and mistakes are not replicated. In the context of evaluating TECS you'll be aiming to gather evidence that will support or refute ongoing use of the service. This may be through, for example:

* determining whether the service detects a person's health problems or initial signs of deterioration at an earlier stage
* establishing whether the service helps to trigger appropriate patient or service user actions or rapid clinician or carer responses which avoid unnecessary health or social care usage
* estimating costs and savings to NHS or social care funds
* identifying ways that the service could be improved in the future.

What will you evaluate?

TECS include a vast variety of services, from online consultations (e.g. www. pushdoctor.co.uk/) and apps (e.g. http://chronicpainapp.com/) through to mobile phone messaging systems (e.g. simple telehealth www.simple.uk.net/), but the approach to evaluation of any of these services is generally similar. Broadly there is a number of features of a service that you may choose to evaluate: (any or all of) costs, benefits, risks and challenges. The *Digital Inclusion Outcomes Framework*[5] is worth referring to as it has been developed for, among other things, supporting local evaluation of generic digital services. It outlines digital (including access, use, confidence, skills and motivation), economic and health and social outcomes and specific, measurable indicators which have been designed to track progress towards the outcomes.[5] This framework has been designed to be adapted and extended to promote relevance across a broad range of technologies. More specifically for health and social care services, the outcomes of your evaluation (depending on the aims of your service) may focus on the following.

1. **Enhanced patient autonomy** – do patients understand their long-term condition better or the adverse effects of their lifestyle habits? Has the patient remained independent at home rather than entering a continuing care home? Has medication or other treatment been titrated against an agreed care plan?

2. **Impact on healthcare usage** – the impact of your TECS may simply be fewer or no avoidable hospital admissions or trips to A&E; less wastage of medications as patients take them regularly at the right dose or right time; fewer follow-up visits to a GP or any other overseeing care professional as remote transmission of person's vital signs or other bodily measures safely substitutes for face-to-face clinic visits, with at least as good quality of care. However, there is a risk, even with a successful service, in terms of clinical outcomes, that your service may result in increased healthcare use, at least in the early stages; for example, patients have extra appointments to set up the technology or troubleshoot problems. See www.nuffieldtrust.org.uk/publica tions/impact-telehealth-use-hospital-care-and-mortality for a recent relevant report on the impact of telehealth.

3. **Breadth of patient or service user engagement** – your service may have been developed to provide efficient delivery of healthcare to allow a greater number of people to receive services or to reach a different patient group to those using traditional settings. In these contexts, simply assessing clinical outcomes and healthcare usage would not present a complete illustration of the impact of your service. For example, hard to reach populations may have worse control and higher levels of unscheduled hospital use and thus may have 'worse' clinical outcomes from your service than other users or users of traditional care. Such results may undermine the achievements of your service even if they represent improved outcomes for these patients than would have occurred without it. So consider carefully how to capture this type of information (e.g. patient or service user report, examination of health or social care usage), or at least explicitly mention it as an explanation of findings when applicable.

4. **Impact on clinical outcomes** – real (or close to real) time monitoring of vital signs and test results may enable more rapid titration of medication (e.g. antihypertensive drugs) or initiation of medication to prevent deterioration

when telehealth responses indicate an exacerbation of a health condition (e.g. rescue medication for COPD; or step up/step down dose regimes for asthma). It is possible, however, in the case where you are trying to make delivery of services more efficient that rather than looking for improved clinical outcomes, you are instead going to be looking for lack of a reduction in outcomes (non-inferiority) and an absence of risk to judge safety.

5. **Patient or service user satisfaction** – patients, their family or carers may have a more positive experience of care when they are trusted to measure aspects of their health (e.g. blood pressure, oxygen saturations, weight) or well-being (e.g. mental health scores) and relay reliable responses to the responsible care professionals in their own time. This may lead to a greater understanding of their condition and factors that affect their well-being. Also, they may value regular contact with health or social care services even if this is automated.[6]

6. **Patient motivation** – your service may be designed to promote or support patient motivation, for example, for them to persist with smoking cessation, weight management and an alcohol-free lifestyle – through regular encouragement and questioning – so that individuals do not give up on tough days. This might be via improved education and feedback about the impact of changes made. Even before changes have been made or clinical outcomes have improved, people may have been engaged in your service and moved towards taking action. Therefore, if your service is designed to improve motivation, you will need to consider collecting information about a shift in a person's position towards the final goal, rather than simply assessing absolute achievement of this.

7. **Patient engagement** – such engagement may be linked with satisfaction and clinical outcomes. The relationship and measurement of adherence to service protocols and extent of time engaging with the service will provide some information about the acceptability of the service to patients. One benefit of collecting patient engagement data is that information may be obtainable automatically from the technology platform being used to deliver the service. However, the relationship between engagement and the 'success' of your service will not be exact; for example, patients may engage with your TECS for a short time, feel that they have been adequately upskilled to manage their long-term condition and then stop using it but still continue their learnt changes in behaviour.

8. **Person-centred approach** – in most cases evaluation should include a focus on the elements of care and support and treatment that matter most to the patient, family and carers. You might gather qualitative and quantitative data to measure their experience of care based on principles of person-centred care:
   - dignity, compassion and respect
   - coordination of care, support or treatment
   - personalised care, support or treatment

- support for a person to recognise and develop their own strengths and abilities to live an independent and fulfilling life.[7]

9. **Professionals' acceptance of the technology** – while some TECS are a positive solution to a well-known problem, others may evoke negativity from (potential) care professional users. Such a response may be provoked for a variety of reasons; for example, lack of identified need, perceived threats to time delivering care, patient safety and patient–doctor relationship, frustration with frequent changes to service delivery and its associated disruption, and lack of familiarity with the technology. Professionals' acceptance (intentional or voluntary use[8]) of a TECS can be assessed by a tool such as the (modified) technology acceptance model (TAM).[9] Assessing professionals' acceptance is particularly worth doing if their engagement is key to the success of your service, as it can help to identify the reasons why some (potential) users did not engage with the TECS or subsequently disengaged. While various iterations of the TAM exist and the model does not always exactly explain professionals' use of TECS, the TAM is valuable as its core components focus on key beliefs about (factors influencing) professionals' acceptance: their beliefs about the use and ease of use of the service, and thus their subsequent intention to use the service.[8–10] It is also specific to the context of technology, which may improve the accuracy of explaining behaviour and set it apart from other more generic behavioural models (e.g. the theory of planned behaviour),[8,10] and has been used to investigate acceptance of a variety of technologies in the healthcare setting.[8] Factors relating to the TAM can be investigated using cross-sectional questionnaires;[10,11] professional engagement or use of the service may be established through the proportion of appropriate patients who are offered the service.

EXAMPLE 16.2 The experience of a TECS facilitator

Chris Chambers

'In the West Midlands we have been trying to drive the use of simple telehealth in three areas – Sandwell and Birmingham, Coventry and Rugby, and Staffordshire. The response from some of these areas has been patchy, as it is a process of change, and it takes time for individual clinical leaders to appreciate the benefits, and then persuade colleagues to join in, especially when the work is based on a project which is time limited, and would need its own financial stream in the future. So it has taken time for trusts and CCGs who have little or no experience of using this type of technology to actually start spreading the word. However, Sandwell and West Birmingham have developed their own diabetes protocols, and are working on rheumatology and asthma. They are also keen to collaborate with a trust in the North East of England and North Cumbria that is using simple telehealth for gestational diabetes. Pharmacists in Staffordshire are starting to get involved with using simple telehealth for integrated applications between GPs and pharmacists.

To reinforce future and continuing funding, trusts and CCGs require evaluation of the benefits, and evaluation is part of the current programme. However, this is very difficult, as what we really want to do is to look at the usage of healthcare by patients who are using simple telehealth to see whether the interventions make a difference. For this we need comparisons of healthcare usage over time, and permission to extract data from different sources – GP surgeries, hospitals, etc. So we have included a request in the patient consent form for patients to give their permission to use their data anonymously; that has been endorsed by relevant Caldicott Guardians of the NHS organisations. Even with this, the task seems formidable, and for quick results we may have to rely on individual feedback from patients to simple questions about whether the technology has helped them to: gain better breathing control; remember to take their medication; or feel confident in managing their condition. We are about to survey clinicians as well about their experience of using Flo for their patients. But I know that the trusts and CCGs will want more valid and reliable data. Yet they don't seem to be able or motivated to help us gather that data on healthcare usage.'

10. **Professional satisfaction with service delivery and support** – slightly different to the acceptance of the technology itself is the professionals' satisfaction with how the service was delivered and supported. It may be particularly important to differentiate professional satisfaction with the support and delivery of the service if the service has failed to identify whether it is the technology or the associated infrastructure that needs to be changed.

11. **Costs** – while maximising the benefit for a unit cost is an important feature of any health or social care service, determining the cost effectiveness of a TECS service may be very challenging. This is particularly so if the aims of the service were to improve patient satisfaction or education, improve control of long-term conditions, reduce costs to patients (e.g. time off work, reduced time travelling to appointments) or extend services to harder to reach individuals, as in these circumstances the cost savings resulting from the service provision may be intangible or unknown, may not offset costs of the service (e.g. if savings are to patients) or may be significantly delayed (e.g. future avoidance of stroke). However, where possible, the cost implications of a service should be considered. Patient-reported outcome measures (PROMs) are commonly used in health economic evaluation to measure outcomes of health interventions, in economic evaluations of medical technologies and to compare the performance of health service providers.[12,13] PROMs might be condition specific, focused on a specific aspect of health. Generic PROMs measure health-related quality of life generally, enabling comparisons of health across conditions and health services.

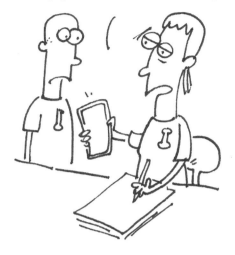

DOING ALL THESE AUDITS AND EVALUATIONS ON OUR SLEEP APP IS SENDING ME TO SLEEP...

EXAMPLE 16.1 (continues) Which elements of sleep-E-head could be evaluated and how?

- Change in quantity or quality of sleep:
  — data collected from the sleep-E-head sensor
  — patient report – questionnaires, interviews, text message questions
  — use (e.g. frequency) of hypnotic medication.
- Reductions in amount of hypnotic medication prescriptions:
  — CCG-wide prescribing data
  — patient medical record review of those using the service.
- Patient or service user satisfaction with the process, specifically educational messages, goal setting appointments with practice nurse, individualised treatment plan:
  — patient report – through questionnaires, interviews, text message questions
  — case studies
  — anecdotal feedback.
- Patient or service user engagement with the service:
  — automated reports from the central server regarding the number of nights the sensor was used and for how long each night
  — patient report – through questionnaires, interviews, text message questions.

- Professional satisfaction with the processes involved in sleep-E-head, specifically the goal setting appointments and ease of use of setting up patients with equipment:
  — questionnaires
  — interviews.
- Professional engagement with the service:
  — proportion of patients prescribed long-term hypnotic medication with recorded offer of joining the service.
- Need for improvements in design or delivery of sleep-E-head for the future:
  — patient or professional questionnaires or interviews
  — experience-based co-design whereby patients and staff work together to improve services based on experiences of care[3]
  — complaints
  — review of the demographics or types of people using the service – are particular groups being left out?[3]
- Costs of sleep-E-head:
  — equipment costs
  — staffing costs
  — costs to patient in attending appointments
  — cost savings – reductions in medications used and days missed from work.

Where do you start?

It is crucial that you match your evaluation to your service provision, so start with the aims you had for your service at the outset. What is the service there to do? Once you are clear about the aims then you can identify the key elements of your service. These may be directly related to the aims of the service or the processes involved in delivering the service. For each element consider what evidence you may be able to gather regarding the service, which may be at individual, service or population levels.[10] This may be routinely collected data via patient, carer or professional feedback or derived from health or social care usage data.

Pragmatically, the evidence you choose to use may not only be determined by what is useful but also by what you have the time and financial resources to collect and analyse. Requiring professionals to implement a (new) TECS service and collect an extensive amount of information about that service may prove to be too great a threat to their time and perceived capacity, and could cause care professionals to disengage, not only with the evaluation but the service too. Also, collection of patient experiences using face-to-face interviews is time consuming in the gathering of the data as well as the transcribing and analysing.

You should develop a clear evaluation protocol. This protocol should detail the aims and objectives of the service that you will be evaluating, the approaches that will be used to measure the relevant outcomes, the types of data collection and the analysis plan. At this stage consider the audiences to whom you will disseminate the results (*see* following), in order to direct what information and outputs you will need to generate from the data. This protocol should be circulated for critique among the team members to ensure that all key features are included; individuals who will be collecting data may need to be approached to check for feasibility too. It may be necessary in some circumstances to allocate funds to reimburse people's time for collecting information or to pay for additional staff cover.

An alternative approach to evaluation is described by Hicks and Boles in their 'comprehensive evaluation model' which highlights the complex nature of the factors involved in the success or failure of a telemedicine service.[10]

EXAMPLE 16.1   (continues): What did the sleep-E-head team evaluate?

Comprehensively evaluating all of the possible elements of sleep-E-head was considered too extensive for the CCG to manage and would have resulted in a dataset that was too large to be useful. Therefore the sleep-E-head team focused its evaluation on establishing whether the original aims of the service had been met and what could be done to improve the service. The sleep-E-head evaluation therefore involved:

- analysis of data from the sleep-E-head sensor to establish the quantity and quality of sleep
- analysis of CCG-wide prescribing data for signals of reductions in the quantity of hypnotic medication prescribing
- patient questionnaires after they'd used the sleep-E-head service, asking about their quality and quantity of sleep now compared to before using the service, use of medications to help with sleep, changes made as a result of the sleep-E-head service and changes they would like to make to the service to make it better for future patients
- practice nurses who were delivering the sleep-E-head service were asked to complete an online survey about ease of setting up goal-based individualised plans and getting patients started with the sleep-E-head sensor, and changes they would like to make to the service to make it better for future patients.

What next?

Evaluations are only worth doing if you are going to disseminate and act on the findings.[3] If your service is performing well, make sure that patients, clinicians and funders are made aware of this to ensure continued provision, dissemination and updating; improved motivation of service team members; and thus sustained patient benefit. Underused and undervalued services run the risk of being underfunded or decommissioned, so their worth needs to be made clear. However, do note that if your service is new, the perceived ease of use versus benefit ratio may be less favourable in the early stages,[8] as patients and professionals need to familiarise themselves with the protocols and equipment to appreciate the benefits (such as prevented deterioration of their condition or saved professional time overall). This issue should be made explicit when communicating your results.

There is a number of interested audiences to whom you should consider communicating your evaluation results. Ideally, for each group, specific targeted information should be provided, rather than using a one size fits all mega-report. Considerations and possible approaches for each potential audience are:

The service team: needs to know what works, what does not work (and why) and how it can improve things should the service be continued. While success stories are motivating for the team, there may always be ways that the service can be improved; feedback to the service team must include, whenever collected, service user data which you must listen to and act on if you are going to improve your TECS in relevant ways. The service team does need to have a good understanding of the actual performance and weaknesses of the service, in order to improve it and help with troubleshooting with existing users. So providing data in a digestible format is key. The value of meeting to discuss the findings is great once the team has analysed the results and has understood the performance of the service, so that areas for improvement can be identified. At this stage it may be worth referring to quality frameworks such as the *Digital Inclusion Outcomes Framework*[5] (mentioned earlier in the chapter) or the ARCHIE framework (anchored, realistic, continuously co-created, human, integrated, evaluated), developed by Greenhalgh *et al.*, which outlines the components of delivering and supporting TECS.[11] Areas for change or development should be listed explicitly within a service team action plan, with details of how each point should be addressed, by whom and by when. Once these improvements have been put in place, you can re-evaluate …

Service users: may be interested to find out whether their experiences match those of others. They may want to know if other service users have gained benefit (which may motivate them to continue) and will want to know if the service was found to be of no benefit and thus they could discontinue their engagement. However, it would be inappropriate to send a technical report to service users. Therefore key messages should be highlighted to service users with links to more detailed reports if available. Dissemination of the evaluation findings to service users can be undertaken in a broad range of formats; for example: the service (or associated service) website, text messaging, pop-ups or newsreels within apps, social media messages, emails, newsletters sent from nursing teams or GP practices etc.

Potential service users: with any service which is new or yet to prove itself, there will be a group of interested care professionals and public who would engage with the service once enough evidence has been produced of its value. Therefore, an important audience is the potential service users. For this group, which by nature includes those with reservations, it can be useful to send out messages about the key benefits arising from the service when it has been found to be of value and also a list of 'frequently asked questions' to present information in a manageable way. Again, the ways in which this information may be relayed can be diverse, through professional and patient meetings, newsletters, websites, social media postings and signposting to further publications and information etc.

Funders: without adequate funding, any service, no matter how beneficial, will fail. Funders therefore need to have the value of the service demonstrated. If you are in a situation in which the evaluation identified problems, but ongoing use of the service may still be appropriate, these 'negative' datasets should be presented to funders for transparency purposes, but the inclusion of explicit action plans will help to demonstrate the necessary changes for future implementation. Funders often have little time to plough through vast reams of data, so make sure that the data is presented logically and clearly, being as concise and focused as possible. Include an executive summary and use appendices to house essential large datasets.

Patient or service user confidentiality

A fundamental principle is that you must not use or disclose any confidential information obtained in the course of your clinical work other than for the clinical care of the person to whom that information relates. All information about the physical and mental health and condition of an identifiable person is confidential; this can only be shared by health and social care professionals if they are a member of the 'direct care team', that is, involved in the provision of care and treatment of the individual patient where such information is necessary for them to do their job.[14]

Exceptions to the above are as follows:

1. If the person consents.
2. If it is in the person's own interest that information should be disclosed, but it is either impossible, or medically undesirable in the person's own interest, to seek the person's consent.
3. If the law requires (and does not merely permit) the health professional to disclose the information.
4. If the health professional has an overriding duty to society to disclose the information.
5. If the health professional agrees that disclosure is necessary to safeguard national security.
6. If the disclosure is necessary to prevent a serious risk to public health.

A patient's consent is assumed for the *necessary* sharing of information with other professionals involved with the care of the person for that episode of care and, where essential, for continuing care. Beyond this informed consent must be obtained.

The Caldicott principles are nationally agreed guidelines of good practice to safeguard confidentiality when information is being used for non-clinical purposes. So:

- justify the purpose
- do not use patient identifiable information unless it is absolutely necessary
- use the minimum necessary patient identifiable information
- access to patient identifiable information should be on a strict need-to-know basis
- everyone with access to patient identifiable information should be aware of his or her responsibilities.

The seventh Caldicott principle is that the duty to share information is as important as the duty to protect confidential information. You should tell patients whom you invite to participate in a survey in relation to evaluation or audit about the standards of confidentiality. You should inform them about the extent to which their identity, contact details and the information they give you is confidential to you, your work team or organisation. Be aware of your responsibilities under the Data Protection Act 1998 as to when you need to seek patient consent. There is a national drive across the NHS to enhance access to a patient's medical records for clinicians working in different healthcare settings, identifying the person by their NHS number.

The information sharing agreement (ISA) is a documented agreement between health and social care organisations describing the who, why, what, when and how details that underpin the sharing of a person's data.

EXAMPLE 16.1 (continues): What was next for sleep-E-head?

After evaluating all available data collected through the sleep-E-head sensors, CCG prescribing data and patient and practice nurse feedback, the team identified that:

- patients' self-reported quantity and quality of sleep improved from baseline, in line with readings from the sensor
- CCG-wide prescribing data showed a slight reduction in hypnotic medication prescribing but in absolute terms the change was minor, and at this stage it was not clear whether it was significant or due to there being only a small number of people using the sleep-E-head service who had been previously prescribed hypnotic medications
- patients were generally positive about the service but reported that the frequency with which they received educational messages was too much and this became a nuisance for some

- practice nurses found the service easy to set up but found that they often ran out of time when undertaking goal-based individualised plans.

The team decided that to continue using the service some changes needed to be made, so the:

- frequency of educational messages was reduced
- recommended time for practice nurse initiation appointments was increased
- utility and potential benefit of the service was disseminated to primary care clinical staff through face-to-face meetings in practices, local GP newsletters and GP educational events.

The results and the action plan were presented to the CCG via an evaluation report. The CCG agreed to continue funding the service for a further year, on the provision that a re-evaluation of the service took place prior to the end of this period and that further funding would only be given if:

- a continued reduction in hypnotic medication was witnessed
- the longer practice nurse appointment times were not detrimental to other healthcare provision (to be established by the next evaluation)
- continued patient benefit was identified
- 10% of patients prescribed a long-term hypnotic medication were offered the service.

The aims of the service, the findings of the evaluation and details of how to refer patients into the service were presented to primary care staff at a local educational meeting. Opportunity was given for practice staff to ask questions about the service, delivery and support and for those practices who had already been involved to share their experiences and suggest ways of implementing the service at a practice level.

FAQs

Q1. How can we disseminate our learning and successes after our evaluation report is finalised?

A. The successes of your service could be spread widely using national media. This is an option to consider if you have demonstrated significant good practice or benefits and your service either has involved a large number of people or has been relevant to a very common condition. Dissemination through the national media would have the benefit of motivating current patient and professional users, raising awareness for other potential users and may prompt other service designers or commissioners to develop the same or similar (successful) approaches.

Lessons learnt from implementing your service may be specific to your particular locality, but it is likely that they may be extrapolated, at least in part, to other areas. So your evaluation can add to the evidence base of the value of different service designs if you publish your results in the public or professional domains. Even if there are negative findings, your experiences may either stop another service being developed if it is destined to fail, or may inform others to alter their service design. Social media can be helpful for giving short messages but publications through medical journals, charity or patient-group organisations and presentations or workshops at conferences and meetings are potential ways of disseminating your experiences.

Q2. What is the difference between evaluation and research?

A. Evaluation is not designed to generate new knowledge, which is research, and usually requires research ethics approval.[1] Further information about what differentiates research from service evaluation and audit can be found on the NHS Health Research Authority website[1] and help you locate your local research ethics department.

References

1. NHS Health Research Authority. *Defining Research*. London: NHS Health Research Authority; 2013. Available at: www.hra.nhs.uk/documents/2013/09/defining-research.pdf
2. Chambers R, Wakley G. *Clinical Audit in Primary Care: demonstrating quality and outcomes*. Abingdon: Radcliffe Publishing; 2005.
3. Primary Care Workforce Commission. *The Future of Primary Care: creating teams for tomorrow*. Leeds: Health Education England; 2015. Available at: https://www.hee.nhs.uk/sites/default/files/documents/The%20Future%20Primary%20Care%20report.pdf
4. Foot C, Gilburt H, Dunn P *et al*. *People in Control of their Own Health and Care: the state of involvement*. London: The King's Fund; 2014. Available at: www.kingsfund.org.uk/sites/files/kf/field/field_publication_file/people-in-control-of-their-own-health-and-care-the-state-of-involvement-november-2014.pdf
5. Government Digital Service (GDS) Digital Inclusion Research Working Group. *Digital Inclusion Outcomes Framework*. Digitalskills.com; 2015. Available at: https://local.go-on.co.uk/resources/the-digital-inclusion-outcomes-framework/
6. Holden R, Karsh B. The Technology Acceptance Model: its past and its future in health care. *J Biomed Inform*. 2010; **43**(1): 159–72.
7. Health Foundation. *Person-centred Care Made Simple: what everyone should know about person-centred care*. London: Health Foundation; 2014. Available at: www.health.org.uk/sites/default/files/PersonCentredCareMadeSimple.pdf
8. Ketikidis P, Dimitrovski T, Lazuras L *et al*. Acceptance of health information technology in health professionals: an application of the revised technology acceptance model. *Health Informatics J*. 2012; **18**(2): 124–34.
9. Yarbrough AK, Smith TB. Technology acceptance among physicians: a new take on TAM. *Med Care Res Rev*. 2007; **64**(6): 650–72.

10. Hicks L, Boles K. A comprehensive model for evaluating telemedicine. *Stud Health Technol Inform*. 2004; **106**: 3–13.

11. Greenhalgh T, Procter R, Wherton J *et al*. What is quality in assisted living technology? The ARCHIE framework for effective telehealth and telecare services. *BMC Med*. 2015; **13**: 91.

12. Devlin N. *Measuring and Valuing Patient Reported Health*. London: Royal Statistical Society; June 2015.

13. Devlin N, Appleby J. *Getting the Most out of PROMs: putting health outcomes at the heart of NHS decision-making*. London: The Kings Fund; 2010. Available at: www.kingsfund. org.uk/sites/files/kf/Getting-the-most-out-of-PROMs-Nancy-Devlin-John-Appleby-Kings-Fund-March-2010.pdf

14. Ripple Community Programme. *Plain English Guide to Information Sharing*. London: Ripple *OSI*; 2015. Available at: http://rippleosi.org/wp-content/uploads/2015/08/Ripple-Plain-English-IG-Guide-July-2015.docx

Chapter 17

The future: what will remote delivery of healthcare look like in five years' time?

John Uttley, Ciaron Hoye, Jayne Birch-Jones

The next five years will bring new healthcare innovations that are even now yet to be considered. With constraints on resources, rising expectations and an escalating demand on services, the NHS and social care system are under increasing strains and unprecedented challenges. Better use of technology enabled care services (TECS) is central to addressing these issues.

So what are we on the cusp of? What is around the corner in relation to TECS? A recent review of how access to innovative medical technologies might be accelerated proposed the case for change.[1]

1. Patients should be given a stronger voice at every stage of the innovation pathway; for example, to direct innovation towards outcomes that patients themselves value; speeding up commissioning of wanted new technologies and models of care and decommissioning those that are out of date.
2. Being much more proactive with making service transformation happen.
3. Supporting innovators in more productive ways to optimise their chances of succeeding with more flexible systems while evaluating risks and benefits of new products and approaches.
4. The NHS should be a more active partner in promoting innovation and be incentivised to adopt new products and systems quickly and effectively.

National strategy

The Health and Social Care Information Centre (HSCIC) has set out a five-year technology strategy that aims to set up the UK as a world leader in the development and use of health and social care apps by 2020. This will create a new architecture for the sector's technology and data services and extend a framework of standards to encourage interoperability and the development of new, digitally enabled services across health and social care settings, such as digital diagnostics.[2]

The plan calls for the implementation of a common digital platform for integrated healthcare, and the use of new applications and devices, such as wearable technology to improve delivery of services. By 2020, the UK should be recognised globally as a most attractive place to launch radically new ways of using data, information and digital technologies to deliver fundamentally different forms of care. The strapline is 'Paper free at the point of care' (PF@POC); with local digital roadmaps underpinning the implementation of the strategy. All major NHS organisations will help to build the required infrastructure once they have reviewed their current digital maturity and capabilities.

A seamless integrated care service requires seamless IT. There should be compatible IT systems that connect as patients move between GPs, hospital consultants, care workers, nurses, therapists, pharmacists and others – if integrated health and social care is to be a reality. Digitising referral forms with templates agreed by all local health and social care organisations should allow patient identifiable data to be immediately transferred, reducing delays in patient flow along care pathways, ensuring that patients need only tell their medical story once. Improvements to the underlying NHS infrastructure should include email connectivity too.

The future is already here

There are currently 7 billion or so active mobile phone subscriptions worldwide, the equivalent of 96% of the global population.[3] Sportwatch sensors which continuously record and passively capture vital signs have the equivalent of intensive care unit monitoring on a person's wrist, without the costs and risk of infections and other complications. Hospitals of the future are likely to become roomless data surveillance centres for remote patient monitoring.

Self-tracking is becoming the norm; for example, in 2012, a 'United Sniffles of America flu map' was created using Facebook and Twitter which was six times quicker than the Centers for Disease Control and Prevention at predicting outbreaks (http://journalisted.com/article/4vg4v) of flu.

In the same year, a company created a prototype sensor: a studded sports bra to be worn by women for just half a day which could make breast cancer screening both easier and more effective.

The possibilities that adoption and dissemination of TECS could bring

With an ever increasing extent of TECS already being implemented and evaluated and new products being developed and entering the market, we have not fully exploited and mainstreamed the resources to which we already have access. Many clinicians say that they are not prepared to utilise technologies without substantive evidence in the form of randomised control trials. These take years and large budgets to undertake and, particularly in this market, will be outdated by the time results are published. Other more timely evaluation methods need to be employed, with results and lessons learned feeding into the development of next generation TECS. And clinicians need to accept that there is no robust research evidence for much of the care they provide now.

The future of sensors will also include passive data gathering, meaningful interpretation and those which are internally attached to body organs. These will include:

- necklaces that can monitor heart function and check the amount of fluid in your lungs, contact lenses that can track your glucose levels or your eye pressure and headbands that can capture brain waves
- wireless and wearable sensors that can track vital signs without touch
- sensors that will be able to monitor exposure to radiation, air pollution or pesticides in food
- medications that will be digitised to ensure that they have been taken as prescribed
- socks and shoes to analyse gait; for instance, to help a patient with Parkinson's disease understand the effectiveness of their medication; or tell a carer whether an elderly family member is unsteady and at risk of falling.

It isn't just hospital rooms which are being transformed; so are their labs. Smartphone attachments will soon be available that enable you to perform a variety of routine lab tests via your phone. Blood electrolytes; liver, kidney and thyroid function; analysis of breath, sweat and urine will all be checkable with small samples in little labs that plug directly into smartphones, enabling self-testing at a fraction of the current cost.

In the next 10 years monitoring of almost every organ will be possible. Nano-sensors will be available to embed in your bloodstream or be fixed to a micro-stent in a tiny blood vessel, keeping your blood under constant surveillance for the identification of cancer, autoimmune attacks and damage to artery walls which can lead to hearts attacks and strokes.

Mental health also has significant benefits to gain from smartphones which can quantify someone's state of mind through tone and inflection of voice, facial expression, breathing pattern, heart rate, galvanic skin response, blood pressure and even the frequency and content of emails and texts.

'Virtual psychiatrists' have provided an unexpected advantage given that people have shown that they are more willing to disclose their inner thoughts to a computer avatar or virtual human than to a real person. With the ability for computers to quantify moods and even provide virtual counselling, this could address the lack of mental health professionals and offer an insight into new approaches to improving people's mental health.

EXAMPLE 17.1   Thinking city-wide: setting up an intelligent city

This example, outlines some of the issues that face the NHS and social care as a whole, including thinking on a city-wide basis if setting up TECS at scale. The example focuses on Birmingham City. It describes what technological infrastructures could be employed to address not only the immediate issues in health and social care, but also to provide a foundation for future initiatives. It attempts to outline the anticipated financial implications both at inception and throughout the proposed five year lifespan, definition of proposed project methodology, early risks and issues identified and mitigating actions.

The context and need for change can be summarised in two statements:

1. The nature of healthcare is changing to a far more consumerist position. Citizens have an expectation that they can access healthcare and care professionals when and where they need them, rather than when they happen to be available or when their general practices are open or the social care offices are functioning.
2. The population of the UK and specifically Birmingham is increasingly diverse, which means that traditional methods of communication are failing. Different cultural and language requirements mean that a single method of communication no longer suffices.

These two issues could be resolved by implementing three technological systems that have individual benefits and a symbiotic relationship, as follows:

1. Introduction of a city-wide Wi-Fi solution, with both a public and private face. A public face will allow citizens to access and interact with their care records. Patients could, for example, book appointments, request prescriptions or even check their test results. The private facing connectivity would facilitate clinicians with access to systems in any location in the city, allowing significant change to the essential nature of the patient–clinician relationship, removing the need for paper records and improving the quality of clinical treatment that citizens receive.
2. Inclusion of a patient facing 'app' would provide easy patient access to agreed services and information. This would provide a governance framework and set foundations for the future of a patient-centred service design.
3. Placement of a network of digital signs, inside and outside of healthcare locations, as well as high traffic locations in the city. Utilisation of tools such as Google Translate, combined with city demographic data, would allow messages to be posted to the populace. However, unlike current methods, disparate messages

could then be posted to disparate sections of the city at any one time. Information about other healthcare services and out of hours' provision could be made available at key locations in the city, with the aim being to change citizens' behaviour and patient demand within the system.

Figure 17.1 relays the plan at a very broad high level to generate the potential impact on the health economy if the city was stratified.

Impact on patient engagement

We cannot rely on existing dated methods of engaging and communicating to the population. If we are to truly succeed in delivering a world class, integrated health and social care platform, we must re-imagine the position that the citizen holds within it. Citizens must be placed as stakeholders within their health or social care journey, rather than solely as service users. Involving citizens in access to provision of their care has direct benefits in ownership and education, empowering the citizen to understand their requirements and take more control of their situation.

The engagement effect is continued through the ability of service professionals to access appropriate patient or service user records wherever their interactions may happen to occur.

This truly is a right time, right place and more importantly *right now* system. Allowing service professionals and service users to access appropriate records when *they need* rather than when *they can* is key to reforming the current approach taken by the public sector.

Impact on communications

Effective communication is pivotal to any successful service platform, ensuring that all stakeholders are aware of key information and messages. But currently

---

EXAMPLE 17.2 Using social networks to help a town run more smoothly

The mayor of the town of Jun in southern Spain has arranged for all residents to be able to tweet the town's employees to request help, such as from the police, so that they might report problems such as broken street lights. The mayor describes responding to around 85 local people a day, ensuring that local people's voices are directly heard. The mayor believes that strengthening social media networks has allowed citizens to integrate and socialise more.

See www.theguardian.com/technology/2015/jul/02/twitter-jun-spain-bureaucracy-local-government

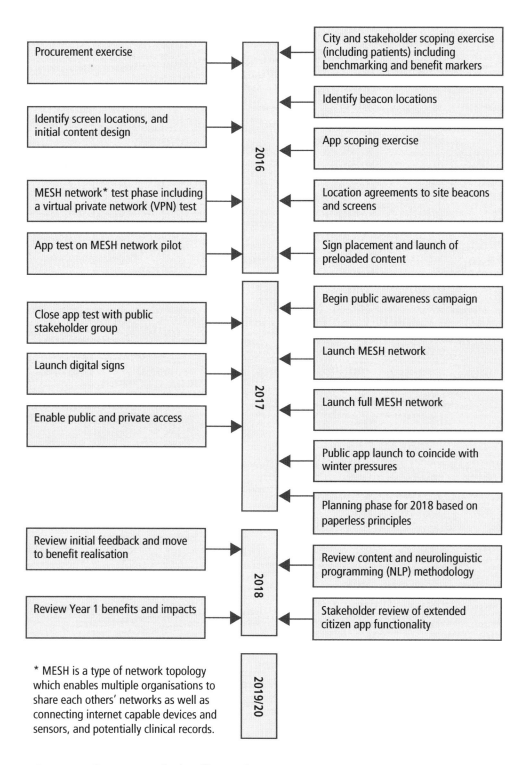

FIGURE 17.1 Progress to the intelligent city

the public sector still places undue reliance on outmoded and outdated paper-based communications. This city-wide project proposes radical and long overdue changes, bringing the public sector in line with the commercial world. It involves harnessing the power of the digital age to get relevant messages to the right target audience – as in the case study of Example 17.2: the right message to the right people at the right time.

Impact on public health and public behaviour

Public health has long been accepted as a necessary requirement to tackle the growing health and social needs of our population, but has time and again not been handed the tools that it so clearly requires to communicate. Use of effective communication methods that place the right message in the mind of the right person at the right time is essential if we are to change public behaviour. We have for a long time laboured under the mistaken principles – for example, that placing public health posters within GP practices educates the population.

If we are in fact earnest about spreading these messages it cannot be left as a dull message on the wall of 'my healthcare establishment', but instead a vibrant and engaging invitation within my daily life. Digital signage is a way to interact with everyone. It can be used to advise citizens who do not use healthcare services about the benefits of a flu vaccination or a healthy diet in a way that appeals and relates to them, for instance.

Impact on long-term conditions

Very few of us can claim to truly understand or communicate about a health condition after a series of 10-minute briefings, yet this is what we expect of clinicians and citizens. We expect them to communicate and understand complex statements regarding their current health problems within the window of a 10-minute consultation. If you think of the relationship between student and teacher, it is expected that time is spent outlining the problem and giving it context before examining the solution. However, in the NHS it is considered acceptable for a service professional to both explain and manage a condition within this time frame.

'Give a man a fish and he will eat for a day; teach a man to fish and you feed him for a lifetime.' The same can be said to be true about long-term conditions. It should be an expectation that people can be provided with the information they need to manage their conditions with the advice they need to live life healthily and happily. Pre-diabetes, for instance, can often be reversed and the risk of developing Type 2 diabetes is reduced by 60%, simply through losing a moderate amount of weight; adopting a healthy, balanced diet; and increasing physical activity levels.

Impact of understanding

Understanding is the first step to expectation. If a citizen understands the nature of their situation or condition, this will set their expectation of how they should be treated. There are some cases where it is appropriate to go directly to hospital, but this step is used as a first action by many due to that lack of understanding. The perception that hospital is the best place to be treated is one that pervades our society. The consumerist expectation that the biggest and most expensive solution must be the best is one that pervades our daily lives.

Citizens should understand not only their own situation but also that in health and social care. The various impacts relayed here collectively lead to understanding. Understanding sets expectation, and expectation governs demand. That understanding both as service providers and as service recipients will allow us to redefine those services.

Impact on finance

The public sector must drive financial efficiencies if it is to survive. Benefits of improved public health campaigns may take five to ten years to be realised, but this preventative approach will hold large-scale impacts on long-term affordability.

In the medium term there are cost-releasing benefits around improved compliance with treatment and regimes based on improved understanding and awareness of conditions.

Short-term gains can be made in changing behaviour, to move urgent care demand from A&E units, to out of hours providers.

Benefits realisation

Table 17.1 attempts to give a high-level overview of some of the benefits that could be realised and how they relate to the wider strategy.

TABLE 17.1 Overview of benefits of TECS

Benefit	Cash releasing	Non-quantifiable	Quality, innovation, productivity and partnership (QIPP)
Change in use of urgent care services away from A&E	X		X
Improved uptake of public health campaigns		X	X
Better management of long-term conditions	X		X
Improved patient experience		X	X
Longer life expectancy		X	
Reducing trends in prevalence rates of long-term conditions	X	X	X

The future development of healthcare: with genomics

The 'intelligent city' (*see* Figure 17.1) summary above describes the innovations that will be implemented in the next two to three years which will invariably be adopted more widely across the NHS and social care as a whole. So what other technologies are going to revolutionise today's healthcare? What will really happen and not just be talked about and options debated?

There is a national drive to person-centred care. We have for many years in the NHS held the notion that patient-centred care is what we should aim for, but this has been more around treating the patient and regarding the individual conditions as separate and unrelated pathways when the commonality is the single patient being treated. Patient-centred care is about to be redefined with the implementation of the NHS Genome Project. This could be the single most important project that the NHS has adopted which will ultimately change the way in which healthcare is delivered.

The NHS Genome Project looks to map the DNA of 100 000 patients with rare conditions so that we may better understand how to identify the elements of the DNA which cause the rare conditions and certain cancers. This understanding will then form the basis for a future screening programme which will look to identify other at-risk patients as well as provide potential new treatments. The UK is the first nation to bring such a mainstream project into its healthcare provision.

In January 2014, an important milestone was reached; the cost of DNA sequencing dropped below $US1000 per test for the first time and could be completed within two days. This is a vital milestone as the cost of doing DNA sequencing at scale has been one of the reasons that the approach has not been used previously. Indeed the very first DNA sequencing test cost over £2 billion and took 13 years to complete. A large part of the cost is taken up in raw processing capacity since 3 billion pairs of DNA strands need to be sequenced. With the ever increasing processing capability of computers the cost has dropped significantly.

The science behind DNA sequencing holds a number of opportunities for healthcare. First, it can be used to more accurately screen against certain conditions and diseases and cancers. In the current approach to screening in the NHS, this is done by gender, age and family history. For instance, females over 50 years old are screened for breast cancer because risk increases with age. Yet there are many examples every year of females under the age of 50 years being diagnosed with breast cancer. Angelina Jolie underwent DNA sequencing and found that she had a faulty BRCA1 gene which is linked to significantly higher risk of breast and ovarian cancers. With significant family history of breast cancer and the loss of eight relatives to this cancer, she had a double mastectomy. She has since undergone surgery to remove her ovaries and fallopian tubes.[4,5] More widespread genetic testing for cancer-causing mutations would save lives and reduce the amount spent on treating cancers.

The value of DNA screening goes beyond looking for cancers; it can be used to detect other illnesses including long-term conditions such as diabetes, heart conditions, Alzheimer's and other conditions which the NHS spends billions of pounds treating each year. Imagine the power of giving a scientifically based risk report of the conditions a patient will develop and ways in which that risk can be reduced. While doctors give advice today to change people's lifestyles in order to live healthier lives later, a good amount of the population ignores this advice. An overweight male in their early 40s, for example, might understand that there is an increased risk of them a developing heart condition, cancer or diabetes, and make periodic efforts to turn this around. But if they were to be told (after DNA testing) that they would likely develop a particular cancer and by reducing their intake of something would vastly reduce their risk, or that surgery would remove the risk, then they would very likely take that risk seriously. Such information would be seen as reliable, having been hard coded into their genes. And they might well alter their lifestyle habits and sustain a healthier way of life.

The subsequent and vastly more powerful potential of DNA sequencing is in providing accurate medication treatments which will target the affected gene. If you consider the way in which NICE and the US Food and Drug Administration (FDA) currently approve use of drugs for healthcare, the drug company needs to show at least a 75% positive effect on a particular condition. Drugs can be approved for cancers, such as cancer of the throat, but these would not be used to treat other cancers, such as kidney cancer. So, potentially 25% of all patients who are prescribed a drug are given it even though it will have no effect upon them. Herceptin or other well known cancer drugs which patients fought the NHS to receive may have no effect at all on 25% of those who receive it. Consider the impact on the patient who, by adhering to their medication, thinks that they stand a chance at life or a prolonged period with their loved ones only to succumb to the cancer. Consider too the NHS prescribing budget which potentially wastes 25% with no improvement for the patients. The power of DNA sequencing is that we can look at marrying the knowledge of which genes are affected with a database of chemical interactions and the impact on that gene. In this way, we can identify an issue and prescribe a medication which will positively impact upon that condition, with almost complete certainty.

EXAMPLE 17.3   How DNA sequencing can help determine treatment

A powerful example of the potential for this new and emerging science is given by Dr Lucas Wartman, a clinical oncologist in the McDonnell Genome Institute, University of Washington who studies cancer to look for cures. He developed acute lymphoblastic leukaemia which is fatal in adults but curable in children. He underwent two years of traditional cancer treatment (chemotherapy) and his condition went into remission. After two years, his cancer returned and he again started chemotherapy as well as receiving stem cell transplants. Again his cancer went into remission. In 2011, his cancer returned and did not respond to any treatment. It appeared that he would not survive the winter of 2011. He was encouraged by another oncologist to have his whole genome sequenced to see what information it contained. It identified that there were two different tumour cells that were present in his bone marrow. The data also pointed to an unusually high presence of a gene called FTL3. The team then accessed a drug using the gene interaction database and were able to determine that a drug which is used to treat kidney cancer works by targeting hyperactive FTL3. After starting the new treatment, Lucas' cancer has once again gone into remission. This is an early example of how the benefits of DNA sequencing can be used to truly make patient-centred care a reality.[6]

While the promise of DNA sequencing is powerful, there is still much that it will not help with; for example, environmental factors, such as conditions which would develop from living in an area with significant air pollution. It is unlikely to have significant impact on lifestyle choices that patients make except to provide a higher level of risk prediction of developing a given condition.

The future: with wearable technologies

We will need to build the capacity and capability of all citizens to access information, and train health and social care staff members so that they are able to support those who are unable or unwilling to use new technologies. Self-care and public health awareness should begin in primary schools and become part of the national curriculum. This will mean reinvesting in school nurse services, but should provide a cost-effective return on investment in the long term of the children for whose health they care.

EXAMPLE 17.4 Electronic glasses, exoskeletons and seizure identification

Yvonne has had vision problems since she was four years old. After a car accident at the age of seven years, she was diagnosed with Stargardt disease, a form of juvenile macular degeneration. For much of her life, Yvonne, now 34 years old, has lived with a blind spot that covers 98% of her field of vision.

Two years ago, she was approached by a company that makes eSight glasses (electronic glasses for people with low vision). She doubted the device could do anything for her, but within seconds, she was proven wrong (http://esighteyewear.com/eyewear).

The glasses use high-definition cameras to beam images to the peripheral vision, which is often still functioning for many people with low vision. Yvonne found much of her sight restored, almost magically.

'The video of me trying them is online and people have said, "Why aren't you excited or crying?" I'm like, "Because it was like cutting off a limb," she says. "That blind spot had been there most of my life and now it had gone. I was in shock."'

The company also makes bionic exoskeleton suits that help paraplegics and stroke victims regain their ability to walk.

The company began to shift towards medical applications after seeing videos of paraplegic rehabilitation. The suits absorb users' body weight so that leg muscles can be reactivated without significant pain or discomfort. While the technology works best with individuals who have suffered recent injuries, the company is also reporting promising results for chronic problems in those who have been paralysed for some time.

The exoskeletons cost between $100 000 and $150 000, but it is expected that they will eventually come down to around the price of a car, while improving in functionality and size.

New technologies, particularly those classed as wearable technology, will provide real-time monitoring of patient biometrics. Wearable devices are a growing technology that has real healthcare benefits, particularly when combined with the power of smartphones and electronic healthcare records. The benefits of telecare, technology to aid a patient to live independently, such as bed pressure mats, or fall pendants which connect the patient to a call centre, are well established. While it has its uses, telecare technology tends to be single purpose, rarely interacts with other devices and can be expensive, which limits adoption and use. Technology is likely to blur the current distinction of telehealth and telecare so that one smart device, coupled with multiple sensors, will provide greater opportunities to live independently while extending the adoption across health and social care. For example, a falls pendant could be replaced by the patient keeping their smartphone on them, or a wearable device which links to their phone. This device would have a sensor which detects a fall. A smartwatch or bracelet would keep track of movements during sleep, which is the current function of bed mats. Significant advances can be made using wearable technology coupled with smartphones over traditional technology. For example, a bracelet worn by a patient to check their movements during sleep could also be used with a vibration device embedded into the bracelet to send a signal to the patient to move if no movement has been detected for a long time. If the patient falls over, sensors in the bracelet would notify the smartphone and instigate an instant connection to a call centre without any intervention by the patient. Moreover, these events could be automatically logged in the patient's electronic health record so that a referral to the falls service can be made to make modifications to the person's home. Notifications could be sent to family, carers and clinicians.

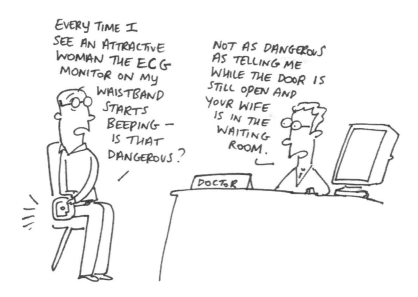

Wearable technology is already tracking blood pressure, heart rate, blood oxygen and even glucose levels in real time. The main limiting factor at present is battery life and common standards for all devices. Battery life will continue to be a challenge which big tech companies will overcome in time, as there is a clear need and the market will demand it. Common standards are important because without them, patients and health and social care will need multiple devices, some of which will not communicate with a device from another manufacturer. This is clearly disadvantageous and inroads are being made by industry itself; with the adoption of health kit standards from Apple, we will see an ever increasing number of interoperable devices. Wearable technology and smartphones are important for another reason. Many people, including the elderly, have already invested in smart devices, which if also used to monitor their health would prevent the need for the public sector to provide them, thereby driving efficiencies.

Wearable makers must therefore learn how to get around these issues by building base hardware products that can be customised and improved via software, which is usually cheaper to develop. Price is often an issue in wearables aimed at disabled users; eSight glasses cost $15 000, for example, because they typically sell to fewer buyers. Smartwatches and fitness trackers such as Fitbits sell for less because they have hundreds of millions of potential buyers, but disabled-orientated wearables cater to niche markets in almost every case. They also often require a high degree of customisability to suit each individual user's needs which raises costs, rather than the one size fits all nature of most mass market products.

Finally, wearable technology and nanotechnology will merge in the future. Nano-health is the idea of a microscopic robot (one-billionth of a metre in size) that when ingested or injected will flow through the bloodstream looking for health problems such as cancer. The power of nanotech is the ability to act together in large numbers to detect issues. Once detected, the nanotech would communicate to a wearable device via radio waves.

Seem too fantastic and futuristic? Then you should look up Google's nano pill. Google is currently working on a pill that a patient would take daily. This pill would put nanotech into your body looking specifically for cancer cells or specific chemicals in the blood which denote an imminent heart attack. This technology, which is in development, is planned to be commercially available around 2021. This further complements the DNA screening process, by actively monitoring for early signs of cancer when 80% of cancers are treatable at early stages. The eventual aim is to replace all tests currently done by doctors with one constant early warning system installed in your body.

And to finish

In order to realise the full potential of technology enabled care, 'technology will need to continue to evolve, providing lower costs and more robust data analytics. In almost all settings, (technological/IT) systems raise questions about data security and privacy. And in most organizations, taking advantage of (technology enabled care) opportunity will require leaders to truly embrace data-driven decision making.'[7] Put simply, we need better access to planned care delivered with a wider primary care team making better use of technology to provide new modes of delivery of consultations and provide improved access to patients' medical records. Telehealth has long been recognised as a key enabler of efficiency in provision of health and social care, with services more focused around the patient and more efficient and effective use of clinical resources resulting in fewer admissions for patients with chronic conditions.[8] We'd better get on with it and make that vision a reality!

References

1. Accelerated Access. *Accelerated Access Review: interim report*. gov.uk; 2015. Available at: www.gov.uk/government/publications/accelerated-access-review-interim-report
2. National Information Board. *Personalised Health and Care 2020: using data and technology to transform outcomes for patients and citizens; a framework for action*. London: National Information Board; 2014. Available at: www.gov.uk/government/uploads/system/uploads/attachment_data/file/384650/NIB_Report.pdf
3. International Telecommunications Union (ITU) ICT Data and Statistics Division. *ICT Facts and Figures: the world in 2015*. Geneva: ITU; 2015. Available at: www.itu.int/en/ITU-D/Statistics/Pages/facts/default.aspx
4. Angelina Jolie ovaries removed: what is the BRCA1 gene, should I get tested and does it mean I'll get cancer? *Independent*. 24 March 2014. Available at: www.independent.co.uk/life-style/health-and-families/health-news/angelina-jolie-ovaries-removed-what-is-the-brca1-gene-should-i-get-tested-and-does-it-mean-ill-get-10129378.html
5. Monti A. As Angelina Jolie reveals she's had new surgery to prevent her 'family' cancer,

it's not just your mother who can pass on ovarian cancer – your father can, too. *Daily Mail Australia*. 31 March 2015. Available at: www.dailymail.co.uk/health/article-3018672/As-Angelina-Jolie-reveals-s-new-surgery-prevent-family-cancer-s-not-just-mother-pass-ovarian-cancer-father-too.html

6. McDonnell Genome Institute. *Doctor Survives Cancer He Studies*. St Louis, MO: McDonnell Genome Institute; n.d. Available at: http://genome.wustl.edu/ARTICLES/detail/doctor-survives-cancer-he-studies/

7. Manyika J, Chui M, Bisson P *et al*. Executive summary. In: McKinsey Global Institute. *The Internet of Things: mapping the value beyond the hype*. McKinsey Global Institute; 2015.

8. Cruickshank J with Beer G, Winpenny E *et al*. *Healthcare Without Walls: a framework for delivering telehealth at scale*. London: 2020Health.org; 2010. Available at: www.2020health.org

Acknowledgement

Many of the examples in this chapter are taken from:

Topol E. The future of medicine is in your smartphone. *Wall Street Journal*. 9 January 2015. Available at: www.wsj.com/articles/the-future-of-medicine-is-in-your-smartphone-1420828632

Further reading

Bland J, Khan H, Loder J *et al*. *The NHS in 2030: a vision of a people powered, knowledge powered health system*. London: Nesta; 2015. Available at: www.nesta.org.uk/sites/default/files/the-nhs-in-2030.pdf

Index

activities of daily living,
  interactive prompts for, 35
activity monitoring systems, 60,
  64–5
advocates, creating, 114
age groups, 7, 20, 96, 106
AIM (Advice and Interactive
  Messaging), 167
AliveCor mobile ECG, 94–5
anticipatory care, 6, 8, 23
antihypertensive drugs, 144,
  232
anxiety
  apps creating, 100
  Flo reducing, 27
  online support for, 109
Apple, 51, 78, 95, 102, 257
appointments
  booking remotely, 7, 99
  interactive reminders for, 35
apps
  and access to services, 101–2
  FAQs on, 103–4
  health uses of, 5, 13–14,
    94–9
  for house calls, 74
  regulations on clinical safety,
    15
  risks of, 99–101, 100
  see also mHealth
AppScript, 103
app stores, 94
ARCHIE framework, 66, 239
arthritis, 62, 161–2
Asperger's syndrome, 35
assistive technology (AT)
  defining quality in, 66
  FAQs on, 52–3, 66–7
  Government interest in, 169
  improving provision of, 51–2
  lack of uptake, 47–50
  in Nottinghamshire, 161,
    163
  and social care, 41–3
  use of term, 43–4, 46, 57
  uses of, 11, 57–8, 63
asthma
  clinical protocols for, 162

  and innovation, 156
atrial fibrillation, 33, 95, 109,
  156
audit cycles, 231
augmented reality (AR), 102
Australia, remote areas of, 11
automatic response messaging,
  9
autonomy
  enhancing patient, 144, 232
  in shared care, 128

battery life, 257
Beauchamp and Childress
  model on clinical ethics, 53
bed exit, managing, 61–2, 65
bed pressure mats, 256
behaviour change, 8, 107, 127,
  141, 152
'big enablers,' 3
Big White Wall, 103
biometrics, and video
  consultations, 81
biosensors, wearable, see
  wearable technology
blood pressure, monitoring by
  telehealth, 30, 32–3, 37
BMI (body mass index), 35, 97
BOLD (better outcomes
  for people with learning
  disabilities), 70–1
brand loyalty, 114
breast cancer screening, 246,
  253
business case
  buy-in of stakeholders, 52
  developing, 151, 170, 171,
    215
  for telehealth in
    Nottinghamshire, 161–3,
    165–8
business plans, 137, 143, 148,
  162–3, 166–7, 171, 212, 216,
  218
buy-in, 52, 162, 190, 226

Caldicott Guardians, 9, 79, 91,
  235

Caldicott principles, 241
call centres, 60, 62, 65, 166,
  256; see also monitoring
  centres
cancer
  clinical protocols for, 162
  and DNA screening, 253–5
  and innovation, 156
  and nano-sensors, 247
carbon monoxide alerts, 61
Care Act, 41–2, 44–6, 53, 136
care at a distance, see remote
  delivery of healthcare
care call system, 60
care management plans, see
  management plans
care pathways, 8, 177, 180,
  183, 219, 246
case conferencing, 70–1
CCGs (Clinical Commissioning
  Groups), 133, 160, 165
CE mark, 15, 93
CFH (Connecting for Health),
  163
change
  cycle of, 154, 155
  tensions for, 188
change management, 49, 54,
  134, 136, 164
chemotherapy, 26, 254
chronic health conditions, 5,
  17, 83, 107
clinical audit, 230–1
Clinical Authority to Deploy
  (CATD), 180, 182, 185
clinical engagement, 72, 164,
  166–7, 169, 191
clinical governance, 6, 9, 138,
  175–7, 189, 217–18
clinical leadership, 160, 172,
  191
clinical management
  enhancing, 141
  level of, 213
clinical outcomes
  impact of TECS on, 232–3
  improved, 17, 140, 144, 192,
    233

clinical protocols, 79, 162, 166
clinical safety assessment, 163,
  179
clinical workshops, 163
clinician–managerial
  relationships, 188
communication
  between management and
    staff, 209
  investing in, 152
  quality of, 96
communication plan, 142, 217
community alarms, 12, 48, 57,
  60–1, 65, 67, 71
community apps, 103
community equipment, 42, 48
community groups, patient-led,
  108–9
community matrons, 25, 32–4,
  37–8, 183
co-morbidities, 33–4, 83, 128,
  141
complaints
  on social media, 114–15
  soliciting, 6
comprehensive evaluation
  model, 238
concordance, 73, 128, 183
confidentiality
  and apps, 93
  in evaluations, 240–1
  of personal data, 5, 88
  and social media, 112, 115,
    117
  and telephone consultations,
    16
conflicts of interest, 130
consequence costs, 151
consultation apps, 95
continuous improvement
  culture, 218–19
COPD (chronic obstructive
  pulmonary disease)
  clinical protocols for, 162
  and Flo, 32–3, 36, 38, 200–1
  and innovation, 156
  and TECS, 17, 141
  and telehealth, 24
  and wearable technology, 95
core competences, 190
counselling, virtual, 248
CPD (continuing professional
  development), 189–90, 226
CQUIN (Commissioning for
  Quality and Innovation), 166
credibility, building, 215–16
cross-boundary working, 188–9,
  191, 209
Cultural Assessment Tools, 188
cultural change, 197, 226

data analyses, 219, 258
Data Protection Act, 93, 241
data retention policy, 186
Data Set Change Notice
  (DSCN), 182
data sharing, 178
deaf patients, 75, 77
defamation, via social media,
  106
dehydration, avoiding, 62–3, 65
dementia
  and AT/eALT, 46–7, 50
  early, 27–8, 31, 63, 157
  and innovation, 156
demographics, 51–2, 59,
  111–12, 162, 237
deterioration, preventing, 17,
  141, 239
diabetes
  clinical protocols for, 162
  self-care for, 28–9
  telehealth and, 30–1, 38,
    170–1
dialysis, home-based, 72
digital delivery of care
  choosing technology for, 9,
    15, 212
  costs of modes, 151
  creating strategy for, 134–6
  encouraging use of, 210
  evaluation of, 144
  involving family in, 213
  learning plan for, 218
  and patient needs, 18–19,
    123, 152–3
  planning for, 217, 221, 222
  practitioners benefiting from,
    152
  productive delivery of, 8, 140
  promoting, 135
  region-wide approach to, 145
  resources for implementation,
    145
  responsibility for, 199, *200*
Digital Inclusion Outcomes
  Framework, 232, 239
digital natives, 74
digital roadmaps, local, 133,
  246
digital signs, 248, 250
digital technology, adoption of, 7
Direct Enhanced Service, 165
Disabled Living Foundation
  (DLF), 19, 60, 66
disclaimers, 115, 131
disjointed care, 180
dissonance, positive, 215
DNA (did not attend) *see*
  non-attendance
DNA screening, 253–5, 258

doctor visits, virtual, 74
Doncaster Clinical
  Commissioning Group, 69
door alerts, 61
dual management plan, 6,
  24–6

eALT (electronic assisted living
  technology), 43, 46–8
eCareCompanion and
  eCareCoordinator, 95
ECG monitors, 24–5, 94–5
EFORTT (Ethical Frameworks
  for Telecare Technologies for
  Older People at Home), 51,
  53
e-health, 23
electronic glasses, 255–7
email, secure, 16–17
empowerment, in shared care,
  128
encryption, 77, 79, 91
engagement effect, 249
epilepsy detectors, 61
Europe
  digital healthcare across, 187
  health apps in, 93
evaluation
  communicating results of,
    238–40
  FAQs on, 242–3
  use of term, 230
evaluation protocols, 237–8
exoskeletons, 255–6

Facebook
  communication about TECS
    on, 129, 212
  general practices using, 110
  health support on, 108–9
  health tracking via, 246
  patient groups on, 109,
    111–12, 210
  use of, 106–7, 111
FaceTime, 7, 73, 75, 78, 80
face-to-face care, 10, 75, 141,
  194
fall detectors, 47–8, 61, 256
falls, managing risk of, 61–2
family members
  and activity monitoring, 64
  coercion by, 7
  including in TECS, 9, 20,
    213
  reducing burden on, 99
fire and rescue services (FRSs),
  61
fitness trackers, 257
five Ws approach, 109, 110
Fixperts, 46, 51

Flo
  CATD for, 182–6
  collaborative community
    around, 193
  evaluation of, 164, 167–9
  FAQs on, 38
  and integrated care, 200–1
  inventor of, 153
  patient experiences of, 27–8,
    124–6, 165, 235
  rollout of, 25–7, 162–7
  telehealth applications of,
    29–37
Flo landline, 31–2, 38
force-field analysis, 221, 222
frailty toolkit training, 214
Furlong Medical Centre, 109

genomics, 253
Google
  Google Maps, 63
  Google Play, 102
  Google Translate, 248
  Googling yourself, 117
  nano pill, 258
gossip, 116
GPS (global positioning
  system), 45, 53, 63–4
GTR (gypsy, traveller, Romany)
  communities, 34

healthcare
  future development of, 253
  minimising avoidable usages,
    6, 18, 144, 232
health coaching, 142
health information, 97, 102,
  107, 109, 112, 134
health literacy, 129–30
HealthPatch, 95
HealthSuite, 95
hearing aids, 49
heart failure
  clinical protocols for, 162
  and Flo, 33, 37
  and innovation, 156
heart rate, 83, 95, 97, 247, 257
H-E-L-P-S M-E acronym, 44,
  45
HSCIC (Health and Social
  Care Information Centre),
  90–1, 124, 179, 183, 246
hypertension
  clinical protocols for, 162
  and Flo, 25, 30
  see also antihypertensive
    drugs

ICT (information and
  communications technology)

see IT (information
  technology)
implementation plans
  adapting for practitioners,
    152
  challenges to, 18
  in Nottinghamshire, 161, 163
  and TECS strategy, 136–8,
    187
IM&T (information
  management and technology)
  see IT (information
  technology)
independence pathways, 26
infections, reducing spread of,
  75
informal carers, 20, 57, 64
information governance (IG)
  and choosing technology, 9
  and implementing TECS,
    177–8
  informed consent and, 179
  and patient records, 6
  and telephone consultations,
    16
  and video consultations, 76,
    90–1
Information Governance
  Toolkit, 178, 185
information sharing, 209, 240–1
information sharing agreement
  (ISA), 241
informed consent
  to automated interactions, 9
  to management plans, 25
  in risk management, 175, 179
  to sharing information, 4
  and telemedicine, 79, 81,
    84–6
innovation
  areas of focus for, 149
  combatting prejudice about,
    211
  environment for, 188–90
  FAQs on, 156–7
  levels of, 147–8
  patient voice in, 245
  skills in promoting, 149,
    150–2
instant messaging (IM), 85
integrated care
  common digital platform for,
    246
  in COPD, 200–1
  FAQs on, 203
  principles of, 199
  and synchronisation of
    policies, 9
  and TECS, 189, 198
intelligent city, 248–9, 250, 253

interactivity, 152, 211
Internet
  access to, 4, 50, 53, 123, 170
  health searches on, 97, 98,
    107
iPads, 77–8, 80, 111
IT (information technology), 43,
  51, 53, 161, 246
iVacc, 97

judgement, in shared care, 128

kettle tipper, 62–3

landlines, 11, 15, 29, 67, 184,
  213
leadership, inspirational, 150–1
league tables, 211
lean thinking, 219
learning disabilities (LD)
  and AT, 46, 50
  and telemedicine, 70–1, 80
learning events, 164
learning styles, 208
Life Sciences Prospectus, 160
lifestyle habits
  adverse, 156–7
  healthy, 6, 133, 141–2
listening
  learning skills of, 216
  in shared care, 128
literature review, 161
long-term conditions (LTCs)
  and apps, 96, 102
  and DNA screening, 254
  and health literacy, 130
  and TECS, 5–8, 17, 170, 251
  telehealth and, 24, 38, 161

management plans
  and apps, 101
  and autonomy, 144, 157
  individualising, 177
management plans (continued)
  shared, 20, 23, 129, 133,
    141, 193
  stepped, 16
  and telehealth, 23, 25, 28,
    38–9
Manage Your Health app, 102
market-shaping activities, 51
MATCH project, 48–9
medical devices
  apps as, 70, 93
  classification as, 153
medication compliance, 26,
  125, 162; see also concordance
medication reminders, using
  Flo, 31–2, 36, 38
Mental Capacity Act, 90, 179

mental health
  and LTCs, 130
  and smartphones, 13, 247–8
Mersey Burns app, 94, 104
mHealth, 29, 93, 95, 103
MHRA (Medicines and
  Healthcare Regulatory
  Agency), 93, 178
migraine diary, 14–15
mobile phones
  and apps, 94
  connectivity of, 11
  consultations via, 15
  and GPS, 63
  and mHealth, 29
  ownership of, 141, 210, 246
  and telehealth, 25, 32, 36,
    162
  see also landlines;
    smartphones; SMS texting
the Modz, 28–9
monitoring centres, 24, 60–3,
  65
motivation
  assessing patients', 195, 233
  sustaining patients', 144
  to sustain TECS, 192, 194
  of team members, 224–5
multidisciplinary teams, 8, 11,
  170
My Health Apps, 94

nanotechnology, 247, 257–8
national resources, 189
networks, improving, 75
NHS (National Health Service)
  and personalisation, 58
  take-up of telehealth in, 3
  working with other
    organisations, 209
NHS Change Model, 219
NHS Choices Health Apps
  Library, 93
NHS England, and TECS, 5,
  59, 193
NHS Genome Project, 253
NHSmail, 16
NICE guidelines, 148, 194
non-attendance, 35, 76, 110
Nottinghamshire
  establishing TECS in, 160–3,
    166–9
  Records and Information
    Group Best Practice Guide
    for, 90
Nottinghamshire Assistive
  Technology Team, 30, 168
nurses
  adoption of telehealth, 223
  and social media, 118

nursing homes
  community matron visits
    to, 34
  video consultations in, 85

online forums, monitoring, 106
opinion leaders, 191
ORCHA, 94
organisational culture, 79, 134,
  188, 195–6, 219
organisational strategy, 151,
  187, 191
overprescribing, 79

PACS (primary and acute care
  systems), 167
paper free at the point of care
  (PF@POC), 133, 246
paper-light services, 159
paraplegic rehabilitation, 256
Parkinson's disease
  and Flo, 31–2, 36, 38
  and telemedicine, 74
'participatients,' 117
partnership, in shared care,
  128
partnership learning, 209, 218
patient education, 94, 127, 202
patient empowerment, 17, 126
patient engagement, 165, 169,
  232–3, 249
patient feedback, 6, 106, 110
patient groups, local, 195
patient leaflets, 129–30
patient records
  access to, 3–4, 6–7
  automatic update of, 256
patients
  communicating evaluation
    results to, 239
  transferring responsibility
    to, 157
patient safety, 7, 9, 99, 182,
  191, 203, 234
Patient Safety Hazard Group,
  184
patient satisfaction, 164–5, 187,
  195, 233, 235
patient stories, 31, 123–4, 164,
  195
PDSA (plan, do, study, act), 219
personal data, 5, 178
personal development plan, 151
personal fitness apps, 95
personality traits, 131, 216
Person-Centred Care (PCC)
  evaluation based on
    principles of, 233–4
  learning about, 209
  national drive to, 253

and telehealth, 38
  use of term, 197–8
PEST analysis, 138, 139
planning process, three-stage
  model of, 138
portable appliance testing, 179
postal services, 79
power of attorney, 179
PPG (patient participation
  group), 111–12, 180
preferred music protocol, 43
prescriptions, ordering repeats
  online, 7
Privacy Impact Assessment
  in choosing technology, 9
  and implementing TECS, 178
  and video consultations, 79,
    81, 90–1
private information, 117
proactive mapping exercise, 164
problem solving, 151, 208, 219
procurement, 18, 51, 179
Productive Notts, 160
project planning, 151–2
PROMs (patient reported
  outcomes measures), 51, 235
psychiatrists, virtual, 247–8
public health, 5, 134, 240,
  251–2, 255
public sector
  communications of, 251
  finance in, 252

QIPP (quality, innovation,
  partnership and productivity),
  160, 164, 252
qualitative reports, 211
quality of care, rising
  expectations of, 41

Rally Round, 99
referral forms, digitising, 246
regulatory powers, 153
REMAP, 46, 53
remote delivery of care, 4, 6,
  70–2, 74, 99, 151, 245
remote monitoring, 12–13, 57,
  95, 246
renal remote care, 72–3
research, and evaluation, 243
risk
  perceptions of, 64
  use of term, 175
risk assessment, 175–6, 180
risk management, 151, 175–7,
  179–81, 185, 217–18
RoboCoaches, 102

Sandwell Telecare Assisting You
  (STAY), 71

SBRI (Small Business Research Initiative), 71, 73
seizure identification, 255
self-care
  and anticipatory care, 8
  and apps, 94, 96–7
  education on, 255
  pathways for, *126*
  promoting, 18, 126–7, 201, *202*
  taking responsibility for, 3–4
  and TECS, 141
  and telehealth, 26, 28, 38, 76
self-care continuum, *201*
self-discipline, 150–1
selfies, 109
self-management
  support for, 127
  and TECS, 5, 8, 17
  and telehealth, 28–30, 38, 162
  and telemedicine, 72
self-tracking, 246
Senior Information Risk Owner, 91
service redesign
  and innovation, 147
  involving patients in, 126
  leading, 215
  support for, 129, 159, 165
  and target populations, 52, 59
service transformation, 70, 134–5, 197, 219, 245
service users, *see* patients
shared care, 8, 38, 127, 198, 210
shared decision making, 127–8
shared management, 4, 142, 156
significant event audit, 220, 221
sign language interpretation, 77
skin cancer diagnosis, 69
Skype
  challenges to using, 76, 79
  and deaf patients, 75, 77–8
  and Flo, 36
Skype consultations, *see* video consultations
sleep-E-head, 229–30, 236–8, 241–2
smartphones
  lab tests via, 247
  medical applications of, 13
    see also apps
  use of, 95–6, 106
smartwatches, 102, 257
Smith, Neil, 215
SMOD (social model of disability), 43–4, 52

smoking cessation
  SMS texting for, 25
  sustained motivation for, 144
  and telehealth, 161–2
SMS texting
  decrease in, 107
  reassurance from, 211
  results of evaluation via, 239
  as telehealth, 24–6, 29, 31–2, 36, 124, 184
  see also Flo
social care
  integration with health care, 35–6, 46, 203
  personalisation in, 58
  remote delivery of, 99
  and TECS, 141
social innovation, 4, 129, 152
social media
  civic use of, 249, 251
  demographics of users, 111
  FAQs on, 118
  guidelines for practitioner use, 115–17
  organisational policies on, 105–6
  patients sourcing information from, 107–9
  promoting telehealth via, 165
  results of evaluation on, 240, 243
  self-marketing on, 216
  sharing symptoms on, 97
  strategies for practices, 109–15
  in TECS, 4–5, 15
  use of, 106–7
sphygmomanometer, 24–6, 81, 141
stakeholder events, 160–1, 163
STH (simple telehealth), 182–3; *see also* telehealth
Stoke-on-Trent
  City Council Telecare Service, 12
  Clinical Commissioning Group, 6, 77, 79, 189
  development of Flo, 25
  social media use in, 107, 109–10
stress, reducing, 76
stroke
  patient support following, 37
  social media videos on, 107
sustainability tools, 168
SWOT analysis, 138–9, 140, 217

tablets, use of, 106
team building, 224–6

technology
  councils promoting, 65
  personalisation of, 47–8, 58
  supporting health and care, 58–9
technology acceptance model (TAM), 234
TECS (technology enabled care services)
  barriers to adoption, 222–4
  benefits of, 252
  and BOLD, 70
  clinical champions of, 190–2
  clinical safety process, 179–80
  collaborative working via, 5–6
  commissioning environment for, 133–4, 159
  communication about, 129–31, 142–3
  engaging patients in, 127–9
  equipping workforce for, 188–90
  evaluation of, 143–4, 194, 229–35, 237
  evolution of, 160
  factors in success of, 172, 195–6, 227
  FAQs on, 20, 131–2, 145
  future of, 245, 247, 258
  improving, 239
  information sources on, 19–20
  infrastructure needed for, 3–4, 226
  integration of, 18–19
  learning about, 207, 213–14
  in NHS, 4–5
  operationalising, 168
  patient experience of, 123–4, 194–5
  patient inclusion and exclusion, 161
  and patient safety, 203
  pilot schemes, 170, 212
  planning for, 137–40, 216–8
  practitioner acceptance of, 140–1, 155, 210–12, 234
  providing permission for, 188
  responsibility for delivery, 199, *200*
  risk management for, 175–7, 180–1
  selecting right type, 17–18, 192–4, 212–13
  strategy for, 135–7
TECS assessment, 18

telecare
    availability of, 18
    cost savings from, 8, 52, 65
    limits of, 256
    technology of, 60–1
    in TECS, 5
    trials of, 160
    uptake of, 48
    use of term, 11–12, 57
teleconsultations, 8, 13, 18, 69,
    91; *see also* video consultations
telehealth
    availability of, 18
    code of practice for, 12–13
    driving use of, 234–5
    frontline staff adoption of,
        223–4
    implementation in
        Nottinghamshire, 161–6
    for specific purposes, 28–30
    in TECS, 5
    trials of, 160
    use of term, 12, 23
    widespread rollout of, 3, 25
    see also Flo
telehealth acceptance
    questionnaire, 195
telehealth equipment, 8, 24–5,
    47
telemedicine
    benefits of, 75
    FAQs on, 79–80
    and renal care, 72–3
    in TECS, 5
    and telehealth, 23, 70
    use of term, 9–10, 69–70

telephone consultations, 15–16,
    30, 76, 79, 91
telephone triage, 7, 11, 16, 25
'Tell Flo' app, 36–7
texting, *see* SMS texting
training, investing in, 152
travel, minimising, 75
TSA (Telecare Services
    Association), 19, 67, 178
Twitter, engaging with patients
    on, 110
Twitter, FAQs on, 118
Twitter
    health tracking via, 246
    use of, 106–7

understanding, 252
unqualified advice, 107–8
UpToDate app, 98
urinary tract infections, 62
user-centred design, 70–1
user involvement, 49, 55, 129,
    218

VA (Veterans' Affairs), 166, 169
values, in shared care, 128
v-connect service, 70, 73
video consultations
    availability of, 18
    benefits and challenges,
        10–11, 75–6
    FAQs on, 80
    growth in use of, 73–5
    informed consent for, 88–9
    patient information leaflet
        on, 87–8

practices using, 77–8
Records and Information
    Group best practice, 90–2
risks and barriers, 78–9
setting up, 10–11, 81–6
in TECS, 5, 7
and telemedicine, 70
virtual ward rounds, 80
virtual wards, 12, 80, 202–3
visual impairment, 36
vital signs monitoring, 8, 13, 26,
    34, 202

walking, safer, 63
wearable technology, 13, 74, 93,
    95, 246–7, 255–8
websites, for TECS information,
    129–30
weight management
    Facebook groups on, 109
    sustained motivation for,
        144
    and telehealth, 161
    using Flo for, 34–5
West Midlands
    ATHome website, 65
    simple telehealth in, 234
West Midlands Academic
    Health Science Network
    (WMAHSN), 19, 135, 200
WhatsApp, 106
white coat syndrome, 30, 76
Whole Systems Demonstrator
    (WSD) programme, 160

YouTube, 105–6, 110, 129